GUT DETOX & CLEANSE - THE NATURAL WAY TO IMPROVING GUT HEALTH

GUT HEALTH COOKBOOK FEATURING OVER 30 DELICIOUS RECIPES

BRITTNEY DAVIS
CRAIG WILLIAMS

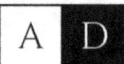

© Copyright 2020 - All rights reserved Admore Publishing

Paperback ISBN: 978-3-96772-039-6

Hardcover ISBN: 978-3-96772-040-2

The content contained within this book may not be reproduced, duplicated or transmitted without direct written permission from the author or the publisher.

Under no circumstances will any blame or legal responsibility be held against the publisher, or author, for any damages, reparation, or monetary loss due to the information contained within this book. Either directly or indirectly.

Cover Design by Rihan W. Cover artwork from DepositPhotos

The Icons used in this work were designed by:

- Freepik, photo3idea_studio, Smashicons, dDara, Kirill Kazachek, Eucalyp.
- DepositPhotos

Published by Admore Publishing: Roßbachstraße, Berlin, Germany

Printed in the United States of America

www.publishing.admore-marketing.com

Disclaimer

This book contains collected information from top experts and sources. All details have been carefully researched and selected but are for informational purposes only. It is not intended to be interpreted as professional medical advice or replace consultation with health care professionals.

Speak to your trusted healthcare professional prior to undergoing any medical procedures, taking any nutritional supplements, or starting an exercise regimen. Reactions and results vary from each individual as there are differences in health conditions.

If you have any underlying health conditions, consult with an appropriately licensed healthcare professional before considering any guidance from this book.

OTHER BOOKS BY BRITTNEY & CRAIG

- Liver Detox & Cleanse

To find more of our books, simply search or click "Brittney Davis" or "Craig Williams" on: www.amazon.com

CONTENTS

Foreword	ix
Introduction	xiii
1. INTRODUCING: YOUR GUT!	**1**
What Is Your Gut?	3
What Does Your Gut Do?	7
2. GUT PROBLEMS	**13**
Causes of Gut Conditions	14
Constipation	16
Hemorrhoids and Fissures	17
Impaction	18
Bloating	18
IBS	19
Celiac Disease	20
Crohn's Disease	21
Stress and Anxiety	22
Poor Sleep	23
Antibiotics	23
Less Common Signs of Gut Related Problems	24
3. HEALING AND PROMOTING GUT HEALTH	**29**
You Are What You Eat	30
Nutrition Basics	31
Sugar and Your Gut	32
Foods the Gut Loves (Prebiotics and Probiotics)	33
High Fiber Foods	34
Fruits and Vegetables	34
Beans, Legumes, and Whole Grains	35
Fermented Foods	36
Plant-Based Eating	37
Drinks	38
Body and Soul	40
Exercise	40
Destress	41

DETOX & CLEANSE

DETOX & CLEANSE	47
How Long Should a Detox Be?	48
Detox Your Kitchen	49
Breakfast	51
Lunch & Dinner	79
Snacks	115
Juices & Shakes	127
Juices & Shakes continued…	131
2 Week Meal Plan	133
4. BONUS: EXERCISE	141
Bloated? Get Moving!	142
The Best Exercises for Gut Health	142
Build Up to It	143
Breathe Intentionally	143
Not Immediately After Meals	144
Check with Your Doctor	144
Yoga	145
Afterword	155
Thank You	159
Resources	161
Other Books By Brittney & Craig	167

FOREWORD

Hi there,

We are Brittney Davis and Craig Williams, and we are passionate about all things health and wellness. Our purpose is to help others in all aspects of building great habits and living a healthier, better life!

You may have grabbed this book because you are interested in finding out more about how the gut works.

Perhaps you are looking for specific guidance on how to best improve your gut health and so your overall health...

... Or you are simply on the look for some great meals and recipes that can help your body naturally detox.

Whatever the reason, **we want to thank you for reading and checking out this book.**

In this book, our aim is to provide a straight-to-the-point, scientifically accurate action plan to enhance gut health. Unlike other health books that focus on overhyped, unhealthy methods to potentially lose weight and detox, we hope to provide you with techniques to improve your wellbeing in a natural form.

Although it's great to read this book all the way through, feel free to skip ahead to different parts you are more interested in. We will cover various topics ranging from gut anatomy and gut diseases to natural detox recipes and health tips. Skip through topics that may not apply to you and get to the things that may be individually relevant to you!

We sincerely thank you again for your interest. Enjoy!

Health
STARTS
in the
GUT.

Unknown

INTRODUCTION

You are what you eat.

That used to be a way to point out that a healthy diet is the foundation of a healthy life, but the truth is, it goes a lot further than that.

What we have learned is that food isn't just fuel for our bodies. It's also fuel for a miraculous colony of trillions of beneficial bacteria that live in our gut. Not only does our food keep these bacteria alive, but it's also critical in maintaining those bacteria in perfect balance and helping to diversify them.

Just a few years ago, most people (including many doctors) thought that the digestive tract was a pretty isolated system in your body. We all believed that everything was fine in our gut, as long as we did not have specific digestive issues.

However, in recent years, scientists, researchers, and doctors have discovered all sorts of surprising effects poor gut health can have on our overall health and well-being. What is even more surprising is that 2,000 years ago, Hippocrates (the father of modern medicine) already attributed all health conditions to the gut.

Here are just a few of the surprising conditions found to have a link to gut health, and more specifically, the gut microbiome:

- Eczema. While not directly caused by gut health, eczema, which is caused by immune system hyperactivity, has been found to respond to rebalancing the gut flora. Fixing the balance of bacteria in the gut helps regulate immune response, which helps treat the flaky, itchy skin associated with eczema.
- Rosacea is another skin condition with links to the gut. Doctors have found that by correcting the small intestinal bacterial overgrowth, or SIBO, they can treat or even eradicate rosacea.
- Anxiety and depression both have links to gut health, and doctors have found that patients experience significant mental health benefits by treating imbalances and gut issues.

Of course, there are also classic digestive issues to contend with, including bloating, flatulence, diarrhea, and constipation. With IBS cases around the world rising significantly in recent decades, it is clear that something is not right with our collective gut.

Everything You Have Been Told Is a Lie

The truth is, when it comes to gut health, nearly everything you have been told and believe about how your gut works, and what is good for it, is wrong. The main reason for this is because so little was known, and nobody knew any better.

We are all told that bacteria are bad and that we need to sanitize everything in our lives. But the truth is, when it comes to your gut, its basic function is based on a delicate balance of beneficial bacteria. When that bacteria, or "gut flora" is out of balance, all sorts of health conditions can result.

Every single thing in your body relies in some part on those microscopic creatures that all work together in a complex and ever-changing environment to process food, keep dangerous pathogens in check, and more. Far from bad, we are learning that these bacteria could be the key to everything from helping heal autism to improving how well you metabolize food and even help with heart disease.

We are told that fat is bad, and sugar is okay, when the truth is something very different.

We've all been told that stomach ulcers are caused by spicy food and aspirin. The truth is that it's another type of bacteria called H. Pylori that is most likely to cause most common types of stomach ulcers.

Gut related conditions, both obvious and less so, are on the rise around the world. A lot of that is because of the things we eat and the things we have been told. Even as medical advances help us live longer and healthier lives, our lifestyle and food choices increase chronic medical conditions.

What's even more surprising is that most of the things we know about the gut only came to light in the last few decades. Even though your gut is so extensive and essential to everything your body does, no one even realized that until very recently.

Because research is ongoing, there are also many gaps in our knowledge. We know there is a gut-related connection or effect but are not quite sure why or how it all works. Which does make getting to a healthy gut a little more complicated.

Thankfully, we do know enough now to outline the steps to good gut health with confidence. So, while research continues to discover more, you can still take steps now to take control of your own health.

Who Are You?

The truth is, if you are reading this, you are pretty much the same person I was. You are likely doing everything you have been told was good for years, but are still feeling tired, bloated, and sluggish.

At one point, I felt so bad, I thought I was going to die. But without even knowing it, I was doing it all to myself.

Even if you do everything that traditional gut health wisdom tells you to, chances are, you have trouble losing weight, you may have skin problems, and you lack focus, motivation, and clarity.

While those are all symptoms of other conditions too, and we always recommend checking with your doctor, there is a good chance that it all traces back to your digestive system. More specifically, it might all be related to the choices you are making that you don't know are causing trouble in your digestive tract.

Everything you eat and drink, along with seemingly insignificant things you may not even know you are doing wrong, could all have your gut health in a tailspin. When that happens, it takes everything with it.

There is a good reason why fitness gurus refer to your belly as your "core". While it may literally be the core of your strength. It is also the core of your health, and if you are not taking good care of it, it cannot take good care of you.

Get Ready to Change Everything

If you thought your gut was just some sort of biological cement mixer that grinds up all the stuff you eat and separates the good stuff from the bad, prepare yourself for a major shift in your thinking.

Your gut actually has a "hand" in most of the things your body does.

Have you ever felt butterflies in your stomach? That is the physical proof of your gut's involvement in your nervous system. In fact, your gut works with your brain to detect and report stress, and it produces 90% of the serotonin your body uses. Since serotonin affects your mood and emotions, it is easy to see how important your gut is to your mental health and well-being.

Of course, that is a double-edged sword too, and there's proof that prolonged stress increases cortisol levels, which in turn increases weight gain, particularly in the belly.

If you needed any more proof that your gut is integral to brain function, there are several recent reports and research papers that link autism spectrum disorders with gene mutation in the brain and the gut.

If mental health and cognitive function were not enough to prove that your gut is critical to everything you do, then perhaps your immune system is.

The acid in your stomach is our first line of defense against everything we eat. It sterilizes food as it is digested and kills most of the dangerous and harmful bacteria.

It does not stop there, though. The walls of your intestines are lined with Peyer's patches, which are clusters of lymphatic tissue, that monitor the gut for any pathogens that might make it through the system and trigger an appropriate immune response.

A healthy gut and balanced gut microbiome have been shown to protect against all kinds of infections, and even cancer.

In short, your gut is one of the most important systems in your body, and when it is even a little out of whack, you can expect to be off your peak.

What You Need to Know

Now that we've touched briefly on what your gut does, and what might go wrong when it's not at peak performance, you probably want to know how this book will help you to improve your gut health and lessen or eliminate the symptoms you've been experiencing.

Think of this as your blueprint to gut health.

We are going to look at what your gut does in more detail and how your lifestyle and choices might negatively impact your digestive health.

Then we will look at the positive steps you can take to eat better and live better, so you can promote and improve gut health.

To make it easier to integrate these changes into your life, we are going to give you recipes, diet tips, and meal plans that are quick and easy, will not break the bank, and don't require a culinary degree.

Finally, we will look at simple lifestyle changes you can make to improve your gut health specifically and your overall health in general.

Before We Move On...

We will get to the really important stuff in a moment, but before we do, you should know who I am and how I can help you.

The truth is, a few years ago, I was just like you. I was eating the same foods I always had, but over the years, instead of keeping me going, the food I ate was dragging me back and slowing me down.

I looked for the easy answers. I tried the shakes, the powders, the pills, and the potions. But the truth is, none of those quick fixes did much for me, and they probably are not doing much for you either.

Crash diets do not work. Restrictive detoxes only leave you starving, so you carbo-load on everything that slows your gut down to a crawl the second it is over. I had a cabinet full of miracle products that did not hold water, let alone walk on it.

So, I stopped looking for the easy solutions, and I started looking for the right ones.

I stopped looking at quick fixes online, with flashy promises to fix it all for one low payment (plus shipping and handling), and I read the research. I read the medical books, and I started following medical professionals who specialize in gut health.

The more I learned, the more I realized that while there are no quick fixes or magic potions to improve gut health, lose weight, gain more energy, and feel lighter (mentally and physically), there are lifestyle changes that can achieve all those things. While they might not be quick, they are surprisingly easy and don't require a big investment of time and money. Just some simple, easy to implement changes to the way you live and what you eat.

This book is not a one-time, disposable detox that makes you feel better for a week and then puts you right back to square one. It is a lifestyle plan that will help you make long term changes you need to support your gut, so it can support you.

I know where you are. I know what you are experiencing, and I know how you can change it.

So, let's get right into it.

Anything that affects the **GUT** will always affect the **BRAIN.**

Dr. Charles Majors

1

INTRODUCING: YOUR GUT!

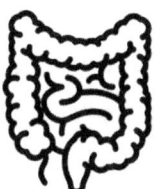

Guts and glory. Gut feeling. Go with your gut. You've got guts. It takes guts. A gutsy move.

Isn't it funny that we talk about our gut so much, but we pay it so little attention? Unless something goes wrong, when was the last time you really stopped to think about what your gut does or what you are doing to it?

If you are like most people, there is a good chance you can't name the various bits and pieces that make up your gut, let alone what their individual jobs are. You will definitely be surprised to learn all of these gut facts:

- Your gut works entirely independently of the brain. It does not require any signals to do the job of digesting food and moving it through your body.
- Your gut has its own nervous system, and there are millions of neurons along its nine-meter length!
- Scientific studies on people with feeding tubes, who do not taste their food at all, have shown that different foods affect their mood differently. Even when they do not know what they are "eating." This shows how your gut even helps put the "comfort" in comfort food!
- Your gut can become physically addicted to different substances because it shares some of the same cells your brain has.

After learning these facts, it is probably not all that surprising that many people call your gut your second brain. In many ways, it does a lot of the same things your brain does, and with all those neurons and nerve endings, it is a huge part of your primal responses to the world around you.

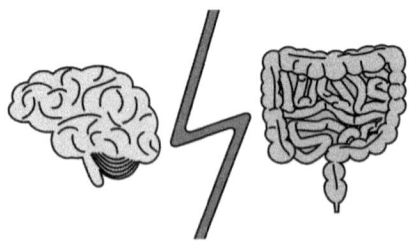

What Is Your Gut?

Your gut is actually a rose with many names (*to completely butcher Shakespeare.*)

What we refer to as the gut is also known as the digestive tract, the gastrointestinal tract, or the digestive system. It is a collection of many organs, starting with your mouth and then going down through the esophagus, stomach, pancreas, liver, gallbladder, small intestine, colon, and finally, the rectum.

Each of the parts of your digestive system performs specialized functions. All of which are essential to the process of digesting food, but also to many other bodily functions.

Mouth

You probably do not think of your mouth as part of the gut, but it is the first part of your digestive system, nonetheless. Your teeth and tongue do a lot of the physical work in your mouth, grinding and breaking down food. But it does not end there. Enzymes in your saliva are the first step in the complex digestive process, and it is here that they mix with food.

Esophagus

Once you chewed your food (and yes, your mother was right when she told you to chew it properly to avoid indigestion!), food travels down the esophagus, which is the long, muscular tube that you call your throat. It clenches and releases in a process known as peristalsis, to move food down towards the stomach. When it gets there, a valve or sphincter lets the food drop into the stomach for the next part of the process.

Note: When people have heartburn or acid reflux, it is actually because the valve between the stomach and the esophagus is not working properly.

Stomach

The stomach produces hydrochloric acid, which not only helps break down food into chemicals and elements we need, but also sterilizes the food we eat.

You might be surprised to learn that there is actually a fair number of "bad" bacteria and other nasties on the food we eat every day. Your stomach, and the acid in it, can sterilize most of those. Although some, like salmonella, listeria, and E. coli, can still make you very sick, so always practice good food hygiene!

The stomach churns away like an acid-filled washing machine, breaking solid food into a liquid called chyme. Which then passes into the small intestine for further processing.

Note: The stomach's part of the digestive process takes several hours, and heavy and fatty foods tend to take longer to digest. This is also why, in cop shows on TV, coroners can estimate "time of death" from stomach contents! Gruesome, but effective!

Small Intestine

The small intestine is where all the nutrients you have eaten in your food are absorbed, passed into the bloodstream, and transported to all the cells and organs that need them to function. This may be why, even though it is the "small intestine," it has a VERY large surface area, thanks to its approximately 21 feet or seven meters length!

The inside of your small intestine is covered in villi, which are small, hair-like structures that further increase the surface area, making the small intestine super absorbent. Much like a towel, with its fuzzy surface!

Liver, Pancreas, Gallbladder

The next step along the digestive tract for your food is the liver, bile duct, pancreas, and gallbladder.

The pancreas secretes enzymes that help to digest carbohydrates, proteins, and fats. It also produces glucagon and insulin to regulate blood sugar. The liver and the bile duct team up to produce and add bile to the digested food, which helps to process fats. The liver then does its own magic, converting the digested food into protein and glucose to fuel and build the body.

The Colon and Rectum

Once the stomach, small intestine, liver, pancreas, and other organs along the way are done with the food you have eaten, what is left is a mixture of water, a few nutrients, and solid waste. The colon absorbs most of the water and electrolytes from this mixture, and then the colon and rectum work together to move the waste out of your body. While that might not seem as important as some of the other functions of the digestive tract, it's worth noting that the waste that is left is highly toxic. If it's not disposed of efficiently, it can cause serious problems of its own.

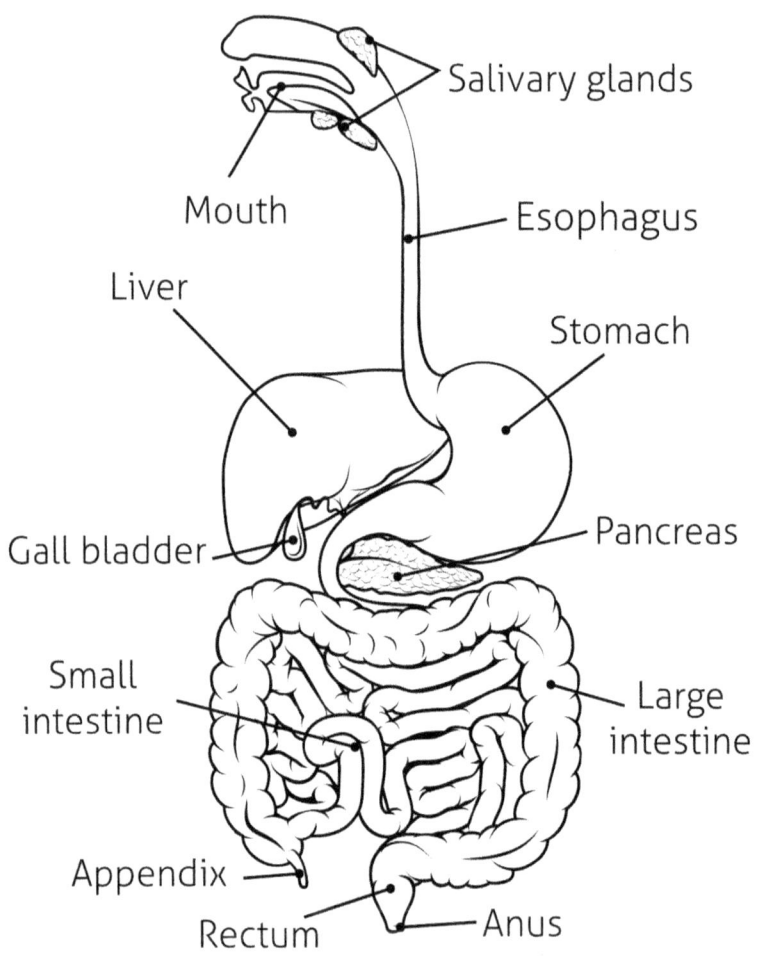

As you can see, while you might think of your gut as one isolated organ, it is actually a complicated collection of specialized organs that perform dozens of functions, all in perfect balance. Your digestive tract passes all the way through your body, so it is physically part of everything as much as it is in function.

It is no wonder that when something is out of whack, you are going to notice!

What Does Your Gut Do?

So far, we have looked at your gut's major claim to fame: *digestion*. However, while it is true that processing the food we eat is a big part of what the digestive tract does, there are also a host of other functions it performs or is part of that contribute to your overall health.

Immune Early Warning System

When you get right down to it, there are only a few ways dangerous viruses, bacteria, and other pathogens can get into our bodies. Either we breathe them in, they come through an opening in the skin or a membrane, or you ingest them.

Because we eat and drink several times a day, and because even when foods look clean and smell "okay," they can be harboring potentially dangerous organisms. Our digestive tract has a significant role to play in immunity and overall wellness.

First, your stomach does an excellent job of literally dissolving most of the dangerous things you eat in the powerful acid it makes. Still, sometimes, things get past that barrier. That is why the intestines have so many neurons and specialized cells that can detect potentially dangerous organisms and alert the brain, which then activates the immune response.

It is why your gut is sometimes called your "second brain." It has a direct line to your actual brain and is often the first warning your body has that something is not right.

Hormone Manufacturing

Your liver and pancreas are part of your digestive tract, and they both either manufacture or control the release of important chemicals like insulin and angiotensinogen. These regulate blood sugar and sodium and potassium levels, respectively.

Without these essential hormones, we would build up dangerous, potentially fatal levels of elements and compounds that we need in smaller amounts to be healthy. That could lead to serious or even fatal health conditions.

A Bacterial Community

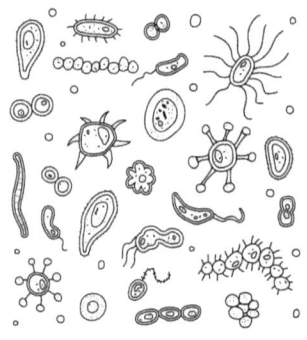

Your gut is home to over 100 billion bacteria that together weigh somewhere between 3.3 and 4.4 pounds (1.5-2 kilograms). They work together in perfect harmony to support the digestive process, and as we are discovering, all sorts of other things as well.

What you might not know is that your microbiome, which is the name for all those little critters that call your intestines home, is as unique as your fingerprints. In fact, even identical twins only have about 20% of the same bacteria in their gut microbiome.

Mood Booster

Last, but certainly not least, your gut produces most of the serotonin in your body.

Serotonin is often called the "happy hormone" because it helps regulate your mood, but it does other things as well. Like transmitting messages between nerve cells, help regulate sleep/wake cycles, and, not surprisingly, your digestive cycles. It also enables you to remember things.

That's not all though, serotonin even contributes to bone density and sexual function! So, while we may know serotonin as a hormone that is critical to mood and mental wellness, it is actually pivotal to so many things we do every day.

Serotonin is so vital that if you suffer from depression, anxiety, or similar mental health conditions, your doctor or therapist may prescribe an SSRI, or Serotonin Reuptake Inhibitor, to help regulate levels and stabilize your mood.

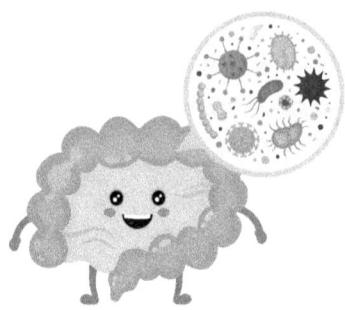

All of the many organs that make up your digestive tract have a variety of functions that are not all related to digestion, but that are critical to mental and physical health and wellness.

Now that we know why the gut is such a big deal in our bodies, it is time to take a closer look at some of the more common and not so common issues. We will also discover how to spot the symptoms and signs that something might not be quite right with our gut.

Every time you eat
is an opportunity
to nourish your body.

Unknown

2

GUT PROBLEMS

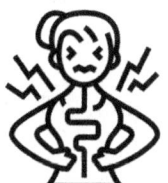

Let us get the bad puns out of the way. If you have a "*gut feeling*" that something is not right in your digestive tract, you are probably right.

There are some obvious signs that all is not well, and when you spot them, you should take action as soon as possible. When it comes to your gut, the old adage "no news is good news" is spot on. But sometimes, the signs that something is a little off is not quite as obvious as you might expect.

In this chapter, we will look at some of the more common gut problems people might experience, what causes them, and what the early warning signs are. We will also look at a few less obvious gut-related conditions and how to spot them.

In many cases, conditions that affect your gut are not particularly dangerous. Still, there are certain cases where you should seek medical attention. Also, most people don't like to talk about these issues, but they are incredibly common. If you happen to suffer from any digestive issues, realize that you are not alone. It's been estimated that around 4 in 10 people have at least one digestive symptom at any time. It may feel awkward to discuss, but don't delay reaching out to a healthcare professional for help and their opinion.

First, if you notice blood in your stool at any time, while this is usually something simple like internal hemorrhoids, it can be a sign of something much more severe. Never ignore this sign.

The same goes for stools that are black and tarry. This is also often a sign that there is internal bleeding further along in the gut and a definite sign that a doctor's visit is necessary.

If you have had loose stools combined with vomiting or nausea for a few days, and you are experiencing fever and chills, it may be a serious virus or food poisoning that could require medical attention. Also, if you haven't been able to "go" for more than a few days, you may be suffering from some type of obstruction or impaction. Again, in this case, medical intervention may be necessary.

In the vast majority of cases where your gut health is a little off, however, you won't have any of these things. Even if you do, most of those cases will turn out to be a lot less severe than you were worried about. It is always better to err on the side of caution, though.

If you do not have any severe symptoms and just need some tips to get relief from mild ones, then the next section is for you.

Causes of Gut Conditions

Often, the cause of gut-related symptoms is external, like bacteria or viruses. In those cases, symptoms will usually be acute and can often

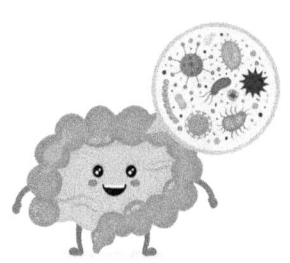

be treated using over the counter remedies and minor dietary changes.

If your symptoms are chronic, which means they continue for weeks or months at a time, or are recurring over time, then they might be related to either your diet and lifestyle, or an underlying condition.

If you have frequent digestive issues, your doctor may diagnose you with a "functional digestive disorder." This is where the intestinal tract and all parts of the gut look normal. There are no abnormalities, blockages, tumors, or polyps, but it does not function properly.

Aside from diet and lifestyle, functional gut disorders can be caused by overuse of laxatives (which makes the muscles of the digestive tract "lazy" and can lead to long term problems), dehydration, pregnancy, certain medications, or avoiding bowel movements.

Whatever the cause of your gut condition, however, the symptoms you experience will be similar.

What Does Idiopathic Mean?

One of the biggest problems with gut health issues is that we're only just starting to learn how much is actually related to your gut and your gut microbiome. In many cases, doctors know that a problem is probably related to your gut. Still, they don't know precisely what is causing it or how exactly to treat it.

When a condition is not entirely understood, or there's no clear cause or treatment option, your doctor may refer to it as "idiopathic." That doesn't mean the information in this book won't help you. It will help everyone who is struggling with gut health-related issues. It just means that there may be a little more trial and error involved in finding the right balance of treatment and lifestyle changes to solve the problem.

Constipation

Constipation is a condition where it is hard to pass stools or where stools are infrequent or incomplete. You may find that you go to the toilet and cannot "go" or that you do, but you only manage a few hard "pebble" like stools and are left feeling like you still need to go again.

Constipation can be caused by several factors, including too little fiber in your diet, poor hydration or mild dehydration, or even certain medications. People who do not get enough exercise can also find that it is harder to pass stools because physical activity helps move food and waste matter through the digestive system.

When people suffer from constipation, their first thought is often to reach for laxatives. Still, laxatives are a short-term solution that should not be used frequently unless under the direction of a doctor. Laxative overuse can make the bowel muscles weaker, which will make it harder to pass stools too, creating a vicious cycle.

Some medications can also cause constipation, as can hormonal changes, for instance, during pregnancy. In those cases, your doctor may be able to prescribe a different medication or advise you about a pregnancy-safe option to get things "moving."

Some people find that drinking warm water, usually, first thing in the morning can help alleviate constipation, as can increasing fiber intake (especially with dried fruits like prunes!) Water-soluble stool softeners that bulk up the stool and promote it to absorb more water can also help without causing too much trouble. If all else fails, there are suppositories that offer quick, short term relief for occasional constipation.

Constipation itself is rarely dangerous, but if you find that you are producing stools less than once a week or are constipated for a prolonged period, and none of these non-medical remedies are working, it's a good idea to consult your doctor.

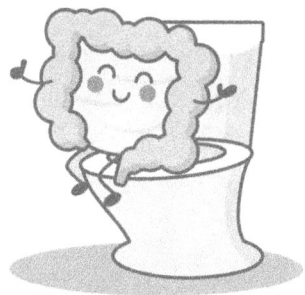

Hemorrhoids and Fissures

They are not strictly related to your gut, but they are constipation complications, so they should be mentioned.

In many cases, people who suffer from constipation also find that they develop hemorrhoids or fissures. These can be in or outside of the body, and sometimes, if you strain too hard when visiting the toilet, they can bleed a little. In this case, the blood is usually bright red because it is from close to the end of the bowel.

While they can be uncomfortable and worrisome, these conditions are usually not severe. They can be treated with over the counter methods and by treating the constipation that causes them.

Impaction

If you are constipated for a very long time in some very rare cases, you may develop an impaction. This happens when too much stool builds up, and you can't pass it yourself. You may feel that even if you do go (and sometimes you can, a little), you still feel "full" and bloated.

Impaction can't be treated with home remedies and over the counter medications, so if you suspect you may have this problem, you will need to visit a doctor for diagnosis and treatment.

Bloating

Everyone experiences bloating sometimes. Maybe it is because you overate at Christmas dinner, or because you drank a fizzy drink too quickly.

However, in most cases, there is an apparent reason for that to happen, and the problem is quickly resolved.

Sometimes, bloating is caused by constipation, or it can also be caused by the menstrual cycle in women. In other cases, it may be as simple as swallowing too much air.

People who suffer from GERD (Gastro-Esophageal Reflux Disease) also commonly suffer from bloating as a side effect of the condition. When you are bloated, you will feel as though your belly is full, even if you have not eaten for a while. It may feel like you need to belch or burp, but the feeling does not go away when you do.

Often, bloating can be treated by simple, over the counter medications that do make you belch. Still, if you have tried that and it did not work, you may need to look for a different cause.

In rare cases, bloating can signify a serious condition, like PCOS, infection, inflammation, or even some kinds of cancer. Still, it is far more common for the issue to be the result of a food sensitivity.

While you should certainly consult your doctor to rule out potentially serious conditions, if nothing is found, you may be told to try an elimination diet, where you avoid certain common trigger foods like dairy, wheat, or soy products. If removing one of those from your diet solves the problem, you likely have a sensitivity to that item.

Bloating can be very uncomfortable, and it can affect your self-esteem and other aspects of your life. Still, it is rarely a sign of anything serious. It is usually manageable with diet and lifestyle changes.

IBS

IBS or Irritable Bowel Syndrome is a common gut disorder that affects the large intestine. It can be tricky to diagnose because there is no specific test for the condition, so doctors have to interpret it based on medical history and symptoms.

Most people who get IBS are younger (under 50), and it is more common in men than women, but it can happen to anyone.

People who have IBS may experience diarrhea, constipation, abdominal pain, and bloating, as well as excess flatulence. Most people who have IBS tend more towards either diarrhea (IBS-D) or constipation (IBS-C), although some experience both.

IBS tends to come and go too, and symptoms may flare up more when individuals are under stress, when they eat certain foods, or (in women) based on their menstrual cycle, because of the associated hormones.

IBS is not only hard to diagnose, but it is also hard to pinpoint the condition's cause. No one knows exactly what causes people to develop the condition. Some theories include muscle contractions or spasms in the bowel, inflammation, nervous system conditions, infections, and changes in the gut flora. Some patients end up having more than one of those, and some have none.

While IBS can be unpleasant to live with, the good news is that it can usually be treated with diet and lifestyle changes, supplemented by the occasional over the counter medication. There is no link between IBS and any increased risk of severe bowel conditions or cancer.

Celiac Disease

Celiac disease is an autoimmune disease that affects around 1% of the population of the developed world. People who have celiac disease experience a debilitating immune response when they eat foods that contain gluten (wheat products, barley, and rye.)

Unlike gluten intolerance, which is merely a short-term irritation triggered by gluten, people who have celiac suffer lasting damage to the villi in their intestines when they eat foods that contain gluten.

Celiac disease is hereditary and cannot be self-diagnosed. So if you suspect you have this condition, you should seek a medical diagnosis to confirm.

It is important to note that gluten is a protein that contains amino acids most people need to be healthy. Cutting gluten out of your diet if you do not have celiac disease will not have any significant benefit, and you may actually be depriving yourself of nutrients you need. Not to mention that gluten-free products are usually considerably more expensive!

People can be diagnosed with celiac at any age. Still, it is less common in very young children and is usually first discovered in teens or individuals in their twenties.

Crohn's Disease

Crohn's disease is another serious bowel condition that affects a tiny portion of the population.

Crohn's is an inflammatory bowel disease that can affect sections of the digestive tract. It is a very serious condition and causes severe abdominal pain, diarrhea, weight loss and malnutrition, and fatigue.

Most people who have Crohn's develop symptoms gradually over time, but some can experience acute onset. The symptoms can also vary from mild to severe or even life-threatening, and they can come and go.

There is no known cure for Crohn's disease, but there are treatments available that will lessen symptoms or even put sufferers into remission.

If you have been experiencing severe abdominal pain or diarrhea that cannot be treated with over the counter medication, visit a medical professional. Particularly if you are experiencing other symptoms like joint pain and unexplained weight loss, you should see your doctor to be screened for Crohn's disease.

Stress and Anxiety

As we have already mentioned, even though they have different functions, the brain and the gut are closely linked. What affects one, often affects the other.

Stress and anxiety, particularly over a long period of time, can have a profound impact on your gut and GI tract.

Many people find that they "comfort eat" when they are stressed, and this alone can lead to problems in the gut. Everything from GERD and heartburn to stomach aches can be triggered by stress-eating.

Stress can also cause muscle spasms, which can take place in the esophagus. When this happens, depending on the location and severity, it can be mistaken for a heart attack.

If you have ever heard or used the phrase "knots in your stomach," you probably also know that stress can affect your stomach. Everything from the feeling of "butterflies" to cramping or nausea and vomiting can be triggered by stress and anxiety.

Finally, stress can affect your bowel, particularly if you have an underlying condition like IBS. It also changes the way your intestines absorb and process nutrients and the production of hormones. It can even trigger bowel spasms, which can be painful.

Everyone suffers from stress and anxiety at some point. We would not be human if we did not. But as with most medical conditions and concerns, the longer it goes on, the more trouble it will cause. In fact, if you are suffering from stress for long enough, you can develop a stress ulcer, which can be painful and challenging to treat.

Poor Sleep

As we know, your gut produces serotonin, which has a role in regulating your circadian rhythms. But what you might not realize is that there are more connections between your gut and your sleep habits than that.

Recent research has shown that poor sleep can negatively affect your gut microbiome, which can affect everything from your mood and energy levels to your digestive health.

When your gut is out of its natural rhythm, it can also affect things like your "regularity," which means you will be getting rid of waste less frequently. While that is not dangerous in the short term, regularity is a sign of gut health. If you are not following your usual "schedule" and not sleeping well, they may be more connected than you think.

According to research, there is also a link between poor sleep and weight gain. Some of this is because we tend to eat more when we are not well-rested, but also because when you are tired, nothing works at peak performance – including your gut.

Antibiotics

Antibiotics are essential in treating bacterial infections, but it's important to note that they are not without problematic side effects.

Aside from the fact that antibiotic overuse has made it harder to treat some infections due to drug resistance, antibiotics also wreak havoc on the bacteria that live inside our bodies. If you've ever suffered from a candida infection or "thrush" after being on antibiotics, you have seen the results of that firsthand.

While treating the infection, the antibiotics also kill off the helpful bacteria in your mouth and other parts of your digestive tract. This allows other pathogens, like candida, a type of fungus to grow out of control. The itchy, painful condition we know as thrush is the result of that, and while you can't see it or feel it like you do in your mouth when it's in your gut, it does happen there too.

Antibiotics are sometimes unavoidable, but if you are prescribed an antibiotic by your doctor, make sure that it's absolutely necessary. If it is, make sure that you increase your intake of probiotics like yogurt while you are taking them, and after you finish the course of treatment.

While some of the conditions on this list of gut disorders, diseases, and problems are serious and will require medical intervention, many can be managed and improved by natural means and lifestyle changes.

Less Common Signs of Gut Related Problems

So far, we've discussed many obvious signs that all is not well in your gut, as well as some of the conditions that can cause the trouble you're having.

But what you might not realize is that there are many signs of poor gut health that aren't as obviously related to digestion. These may include:

- **Mood Disorders**: Because your gut is so closely linked to your brain, when things aren't going well in your digestive system, you may find that you are depressed, anxious, or have mood swings. If you have these symptoms and there is no apparent cause, but you have noticed some intestinal issues,

speak to your doctor. The problem may not be with your head at all – but rather with your microbiome.
- **Lack of Concentration**: Several studies show that gut dysbiosis, or an imbalance in gut flora, can lead to concentration issues and are even linked to learning disabilities in some cases.
- **Skin Conditions, Rashes, Acne, and Eczema**: Your gut is directly linked to your skin through the gut/skin axis. So, when things are out of balance in your digestive system, you may notice the signs on your skin.
- **Chronic Fatigue Syndrome**: Recent studies have shown that people who suffer from chronic fatigue are far more likely to suffer from imbalances in gut flora than those who don't. No one is sure whether one causes the other or if it is merely a sign of trouble, but there is a clear link between the two.
- **Weight Gain**: Yes, if you are eating poorly and not exercising enough, you will gain weight. But there's also growing evidence that when your gut microbiome is out of balance, you will gain weight more easily, and it will be more challenging to lose.
- **Autoimmune Diseases**: Aside from directly related autoimmune conditions like celiac, gut flora imbalance has also been linked to rheumatoid arthritis, diabetes, and multiple sclerosis. There is also a bacterium that is present in your gut called Enterococcus Gallinarum. It is harmless under normal circumstances, but when it multiplies too much, it can travel to your liver and cause another autoimmune disease.

Even if you are diagnosed with an immune or inflammation-related gut condition, your doctor will almost certainly recommend changes to your diet, exercise, and sleep routine. They will probably recommend that you manage stress too, and make other changes that may seem minor but can have a significant impact.

This list of gut conditions is not exhaustive, of course, and other things may be causing your symptoms. But those other things are much less likely, and now that you know what the common causes might be, you can take steps to change your habits and assess what the results of those changes are.

The good news is that you are not powerless. There are things you can start doing right now to improve your gut health, lessen or eliminate your symptoms, and live a happier, healthier life.

It takes guts… but here we go!

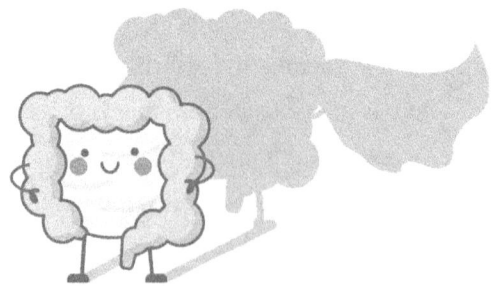

> Anxiety is not all in your head. It's actually in your gut.

Unknown

3

HEALING AND PROMOTING GUT HEALTH

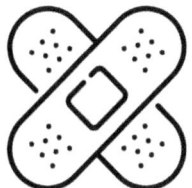

How do you eat an elephant?

One bite at a time.

That is a very old saying, but it is very relevant to the matter of gut health. Literally and figuratively. In this case, it means it is never too late to make a positive change.

Too often, we think we have been doing the wrong things for so long, there is no point in changing our habits, but that is never true.

Even if you haven't made the best choices, may have done a little damage along the way, and are resigned to just living with your symptoms, you can make changes today to start improving your gut health and the way you feel, look and think.

The longer you have been making less than fantastic choices (intentionally or unknowingly), the longer it is likely to take to reach the results you want. But you have to start sometime, and there is no time like the present.

As you can imagine, improving and maintaining good gut health has a lot to do with what you eat. So, a bit part of this chapter is all about foods that are good for your gut and why. But there is more to health than just food, so we will also cover things like exercise, stress management, and sleep habits.

Good health really is holistic.

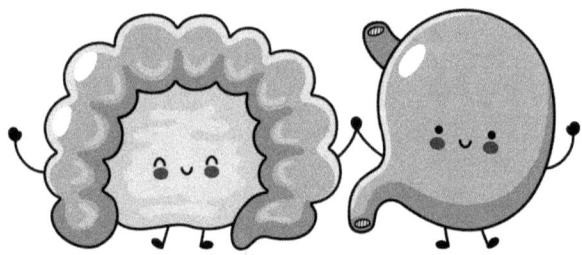

You Are What You Eat

It might surprise you to learn just how accurate that old saying is, but your grandmother was right when she said it.

Whether we are talking in general or gut-specific, the foundation of health starts with what you put into your body. The better quality the food you eat, the more efficiently you can use it, and the less waste your body needs to try to filter out. All of those things add up to better health.

Since your gut is directly involved in the process, that is even more true in this case.

So, while it is always good to have a cheat day from time to time, try to stick to these rules, 80 to 90% of the time, to build the right foundation for better health.

Nutrition Basics

There are endless diet plans out there. Some are healthier than others. Some are specifically designed to lose weight, and some are necessary for medical reasons.

However, when it comes to good nutrition, the basics do not change too much. While we will get into the specifics of gut-healthy foods soon, the following universal rules of nutrition will almost always apply:

- Choose lean protein from meat, fish, poultry, or vegetable sources, and trim any visible fat from animal-based proteins.
- Dairy products and eggs can be good sources of protein and other nutrients, but choose lower fat, unsweetened options, and use healthier cooking methods when possible.
- Eat the rainbow. When it comes to fruits and vegetables, more color is always better. Different color vegetables tend to have

other nutrients in them. The more colors you eat, the more vitamins, minerals, and phytochemicals you get.
- Choose whole grains whenever possible. Carbs are not bad, but refined carbs are not good for you.
- Avoid refined sugar and limit your sugar intake. Refined sugar does not have much nutritional value.
- Do not cut out all the fat. Healthy fats like avocados, oily fish, nuts and seeds, and olive oil are essential to health, so add them to your diet.
- Restrict alcohol, sugary drinks, commercial juices, and snacks.

An excellent way to ensure that you are eating better is to prepare your own meals, using fresh ingredients. If you know what goes into your meals, you have far more control.

Sugar and Your Gut

We will get to foods that your gut loves in a few moments, but before we do, I wanted to delve a little deeper into sugar and why it's so bad for your gut and your health in general.

Diets that are high in sugar have been found to promote chronic inflammation, which irritates your gut. Sugar has also been proven to change the makeup of your gut flora, which can throw everything in your body out of balance.

Sugar also promotes candida growth, which is the same "bad flora" that causes thrush. When there is an overgrowth of candida in your intestines, it actually eats away at the lining of your gut.

While we're on the topic of sweeteners, though, you also need to know that artificial sweeteners are just as bad. In fact, in various research projects, they have been shown to alter the gut flora in ways that promote obesity. So, choosing "sugar-free" foods and beverages might actually be worse for your weight if that is a concern.

In the western world, we eat many more times the amount of sugar we need to function, which is very dangerous in many ways. Because we eat so much of it, we also "build up a resistance" to it, so we can't even taste it much of the time, even when it is present in large quantities.

Of course, it's impossible to completely eliminate sugar from your life and diet, but if you do only one thing after reading this book, start removing added sugar from your diet and making healthier sugar choices. Natural sugar products are always better than refined sugar or sugar substitutes.

Foods the Gut Loves (Prebiotics and Probiotics)

Many products claim to be gut-healthy prebiotics and probiotics. Still, the truth is, like many supplements, you get more benefit from eating the actual foods than you ever will in a pill bottle.

Prebiotics and probiotics have been shown to benefit the gut, and they are actually easy to find in the food we eat.

Prebiotics are undigestible fiber from fruits and vegetables that pass through the digestive tract intact and then ferment in the large intestine. Apple skins, beans, and other fruits and vegetables all contain this type of fiber. When it reaches the large intestine and starts to ferment, the resulting nutrients feed the bacteria of the gut biome.

Probiotics are beneficial bacteria that we find in foods like live-culture yogurt, sauerkraut, miso, and kimchi. These bacteria travel through the gut to the colon, where they make themselves at home as part of your gut microbiome.

Eating foods like these helps to feed the good bacteria in your intestinal tract, and that makes digesting everything easier.

It is especially important to add foods like these to your diet if you have been or are taking an antibiotic. While they can be very beneficial to treat bacterial infections, some (especially broad-spectrum antibiotics) can also decimate your gut flora, leading to problems like thrush and digestive issues.

High Fiber Foods

Fiber is nature's broom. It helps to sweep out the bad stuff and clean out the inside of your gut. Fiber keeps things moving, and when things are moving, we feel better.

Because fiber speeds up the processing of foods (and limits the time that your gut has to absorb fat), it can even help you lose weight (*even if you cheat from time to time!*)

There are several types of food that we can get dietary fiber from. While you should always try to eat a wide variety of foods to get the most benefit, you can choose different fiber sources every day to keep things interesting.

Fruits and Vegetables

Fruits and vegetables are the easiest (and often tastiest) way to get more fiber in your diet. Whenever possible, choose raw or lightly cooked vegetables for the maximum benefit. If you can, eat the peels and skins along with the flesh. Some great fruit and vegetable fiber choices are:

- Leafy greens like kale, spinach, or lettuce.
- Root vegetables like carrots and beets.
- Cruciferous vegetables, including broccoli, cauliflower, and cabbage.
- Sweet potato and regular potatoes (unpeeled).
- Apples, oranges, and strawberries.
- Raspberries and blackberries.
- Bananas, mangos and guavas.

Dried fruits are not a bad source of fiber, although they have high sugar levels, so limit your intake. On the other hand, commercial juices have almost no fiber, so they are not worth the added calories.

Beans, Legumes, and Whole Grains

Beans, legumes, and whole grains are another excellent fiber source, although you usually can't eat them raw! Some easy, tasty sources of fiber include:

- Brown rice.
- Quinoa or mixed grain products.
- Whole grain bread and baked products, or products with added fiber.
- Dried or canned (rinsed) beans, peas, and lentils.

- Oats (preferably steel cut, but most have a decent amount of fiber).
- Fiber cereal products, but be sure to check that they don't have too much sugar or sodium.

Nearly every food choice can be made healthier by opting for a whole grain choice. So, if you must have pizza, choose one with a multigrain crust, or if you feel like having a cookie, have an oatmeal chocolate chip (even better if you bake them yourself!)

Multigrain crackers with hummus are an excellent choice for a fiber-packed snack. Serving meals with quinoa or brown rice instead of white rice or noodles is an easy way to boost every meal's fiber content.

Fermented Foods

Our gut microbiome loves fermented foods, and the helpful bacteria in these products can help boost their numbers. The more good bacteria there are in our gut (and the greater the variety!), the better, so choose any of these foods and add them to your diet:

- Yogurt, but only live culture varieties, and choose plain, sugar-free, and unflavored versions instead of fruity or sugary types.
- Kimchi, which is a type of fermented Korean condiment. It is usually made with cabbage, but there are other types, and they are all available from Asian supermarkets.

- Sauerkraut – the German classic. Delicious on its own or as a tart accompaniment to meats and other foods.
- Kefir, which is another fermented dairy product, similar to yogurt, but with a thinner, pourable consistency.
- Tempeh, which is a fermented soy product. Of course, if you have a soy allergy or sensitivity, avoid this!
- Kombucha, a trendy fermented tea drink that is available in a wide variety of flavors these days.

While all of these foods are great for your gut health, it is a good idea to remember that preparing fermented foods requires a high level of precision and food hygiene. Always buy your fermented food products from a reliable source, who will have prevented cross-contamination and kept the products refrigerated when necessary.

Fermented products are full of good, healthy bacteria that can-do wonders for your gut. But if any foodborne pathogens find their way into the mix, they could cause a severe case of food poisoning, which will have the exact opposite effect.

Also, remember that when we say "live culture," we really mean that there are live, beneficial bacteria in the food products. Like most bacteria, very high heat and freezing can kill them. Try to avoid cooking or freezing live culture products, and make sure that you buy them as fresh as possible and use them quickly.

Plant-Based Eating

While you don't necessarily have to become vegetarian or vegan to improve your gut health, cutting down on meat and animal products and increasing vegetables, fruits and grains can have significant benefits.

By increasing plant-based foods, you can help increase and support the bacteria in your gut and reduce meat and similar products that can be harder to digest. You can also help reduce inflammation at the same time.

If you are worried about getting too little protein, don't be. Many studies have shown that people in developed countries get about double their daily required protein to maintain optimal health. Plus, it is easy to add protein to a vegetarian or plant-based meal with beans, tofu, or even broccoli!

Remember that it can be tricky to balance a fully vegetarian or vegan diet, so if you decide to go fully plant based, it is always a good idea to speak to a doctor or nutritionist to develop a healthy eating plan.

Many vegetarians and vegans also struggle to get enough iron and vitamin B12, as well as Omega 3, 6, and 9 fatty acids. If you plan to go nearly or completely animal-free in your diet, you may need supplements to get those nutrients in sufficient quantities to stay healthy.

Drinks

When you are working on changing the way you drink, don't forget to change the things you drink too.

We all know these days that alcohol can be damaging, and that is true for gut health too. While small amounts in moderation can have other health benefits, too much can reduce the number of healthy gut flora and increase the growth of harmful bacteria. It also has adverse effects on the liver and pancreas.

Moderation is everything, but there are plenty of other drinks you can reach for, such as:

- **Water:** No, we do not necessarily need eight glasses a day, and you do need to be careful not to overhydrate. Still, water is a great choice to keep your gut healthy. Note: if you suffer from serious diarrhea, you should switch water for an electrolyte beverage because you will need to replace the salts you are losing.
- **Kombucha:** As we mentioned before, Kombucha is a type of fermented tea that is sold with various fruit and other flavorings. It is delicious, hydrating, and helps to promote the growth of healthy gut bacteria. Triple win.
- **Herbal Tea:** Herbal tea is great for gut health because it combines the benefits of water with the known medicinal properties of herbs. Ginger, lemongrass, peppermint, and fennel tea are all great for gut health in general, and thyme tea with a little honey is a great way to calm an upset stomach.
- **Coffee:** Yes. It is surprising, but small amounts of coffee are a mild laxative that keep the gut moving. There have also been studies in rats that find that coffee can improve the gut microbiome and help the intestines to contract more efficiently. Which all sounds like too much information, but it is good news for your gut!
- **Kefir:** Another fermented drink that combines the benefits of hydration with supporting your gut flora.
- **Bone Broth:** Bone broth is super trendy right now, and while some of the claims about its health benefits are still being explored, it does contain a large amount of gelatin. Gelatin helps to heal and seal the intestinal tract, and that helps to ensure that everything keeps moving along properly. Always

look for lower salt options, though, because too much salt has adverse effects on other parts of your body.

- **Celery Juice:** Not exactly the first thing you think of when browsing the juice aisle, but celery juice actually contains a mild type of hydrochloric acid. That helps to support gut function and can even help to reduce the prevalence of constipation. While you can dilute celery juice with something more palatable, those in the know say the straight stuff is the most potent!
- **Aloe Juice:** If you thought aloe vera was just something that you find on the beauty store shelves, in various skin lotions and cleansers, think again. The leaves of this fleshy plant can also be eaten (and juiced) and have been shown to reduce the pain and discomfort associated with IBS and other chronic gut conditions. It also serves as a mild natural laxative.

Body and Soul

We all know by now that mental and physical health are two sides of the same coin. It's not possible to have one without the other, so even if you're eating right, you may still find that you have uncomfortable and unpleasant gut-related symptoms or the fatigue and mental fog that can arise as side effects of those.

The secret is to take care of your physical and mental health as well as your diet, and here are a few easy ways you can do just that.

Exercise

Exercise is not just for fitness junkies with a wardrobe full of designer athletic gear. It is a genuine necessity for better health for everyone.

Study after study has shown that exercise boosts mood, improves sleep, keeps your heart healthy, and more. But it has genuine physical health effects too.

Exercise has been proven to help regulate insulin resistance in Type 2 diabetics. It helps to promote digestion and is proven to help treat chronic constipation. Moving, stretching, and walking or running helps encourage peristalsis, which means your gut works better.

Think of your gut as the muscle that much of it is. Workouts are good for all your muscles, including those ones.

Destress

Stress really is the silent killer. It attacks your heart, can trigger strokes and has a direct and detrimental effect on your gut health. It is critical to everyone's health that we all learn to manage stress, and there are several ways that you can do that, including:

- Make time for yourself, where you don't have to meet any deadlines, support anyone else, or take care of family crises. Doing nothing is sometimes the best thing you can do for your health.
- Learn to accept that you cannot do everything, or be everything for everyone, and that it is okay not to be perfect.
- Take up calm, soothing hobbies like reading, gardening, or spend time with your pets. A walk with the dog is a great way to reduce stress!
- Consider meditation, yoga, or tai chi to help focus your mind and keep you grounded.
- Learn to say no. It is hard, but it is an essential part of de-stressing your life.

- If you find that you are just not capable of releasing stress from your life, talk to a counselor, therapist, or even a close friend. Sometimes, all it takes is to have someone really listen.

Being stressed will affect your health negatively, and not only your gut health. The longer you live in a state of stress, the worse the effects will become.

Remember that stress is not just a feeling you have but a biological reaction from your body. Our primal, subconscious minds see stress as "fight or flight" and release a cocktail of hormones to keep us alert and ready to evade danger. While that is okay and even necessary in the short term, it is not good over a long time.

So, give your inner caveman a break, focus on what you can change, and learn to release the things you cannot control.

It is so easy for humans to compartmentalize health. Some obsess about numbers on the scale. Others spend hours in the gym, chasing perfect abs or taut muscles. But what those people tend to miss is that true health is not one thing. It is the sum of all the parts, and gut health is no different. You can't achieve it by doing one thing, cutting out one food, or obsessing about a particular exercise, pill, or potion.

Now that we know what the basic building blocks of a gut-healthy lifestyle are, though, it is time to dive deeper and learn some detailed, natural, and science-based ways to support our gut and all the things it does for us.

Let's build wellness rather than treating disease.

Dr. Bruce Daggy

Detox & Cleanse

DETOX & CLEANSE

"Gut health is the key to overall health."

- Kris Carr.

While the New York Times best-selling wellness guru might have said that recently, she was not the first. In fact, as we have already covered, she might have to concede that honor to Hippocrates.

Whoever wins that battle, though, the basic premise remains: *if you want to feel better, look better and live a healthier life, you need to be able to process fuel efficiently and to do that, you need a healthy gut.*

It is hard to eat healthy, though. At the end of a long day of work, when the dog is demanding a walk and your kids need help with their homework, it is a lot easier to turn to frozen pizza than it is to figure out a healthy meal. You know your gut and body need it, but all you really need right now is to put your feet up and breathe.

This chapter is all about showing you how you can have both, without spending hours in the kitchen.

There are some quick and easy meals you can whip up quickly and easily, that are healthy and tasty, and that won't break the bank.

How Long Should a Detox Be?

You might be wondering how long you need to follow a gut detox. You've probably seen promises about three-day detoxes and miracle resets out there.

Unfortunately, like crash diets, crazily restrictive detoxes that have you drinking nothing but green juice for three days and then binging on junk food because you are starving might do more harm than good.

Feeding your gut flora the wrong things can throw them out of balance, but starving them and then binging will do the same, and probably worse.

The truth is that for a detox to be effective, you will need to follow a reasonably restrictive diet for two to three weeks, but to get ongoing benefits, you will need to make permanent changes to your diet and lifestyle. As soon as you go back to your bad habits, you will start to see their negative effects in your gut and in your life.

That doesn't mean that you need to stick to this type of eating plan every day of your life. Everyone needs to have a little fun (and a greasy burger with a sinful shake) every once in a while, and you'll be far more likely to stick to better habits if you don't feel deprived.

So, once you've followed your new eating plan for two to three weeks, allow yourself to break the rules one day a week. Yes, it's not great for your gut microbiome, but it might be great for your mood, and that's important too.

Detox Your Kitchen

Before we get into the recipes within this book, you should consider doing something, and that is, detoxing your kitchen.

It is a lot easier to make gut-healthy eating choices when you aren't tempted to make some spicy ramen and call it a night. So, before you start any detox plan or lifestyle eating overhaul, you should first take stock of what you have on hand.

While some commercial snacks are okay (and we all have days when only a snack-sized chocolate bar will fix the world), you should limit the number of items you have within easy reach at any time. If you bulk buy, like many people do these days, store "excess" items in a pantry or storeroom, out of easy reach.

Another time-saving tip for healthy eating is to stock up on flash-frozen vegetables, canned, no salt added beans and lentils, and healthy whole grains like barley or quinoa. One of the most common excuses for not eating healthy is that you don't have the right ingredients on hand. While these aren't exactly the same as fresh options, they still have exceptional nutritional value and are quick and easy to prepare.

Keep your fridge stocked with gut-healthy drink options, and invest in some stylish, functional, and easy to clean food containers for work or school. This way, you are not tempted to have a cheeseburger in the drive-through instead.

BREAKFAST

Breakfast has long been considered the most important meal of the day, and there are definite mental and physical benefits to eating a nutritious meal in the morning. Breakfasts are also a great time to load up on gut-healthy fiber, and since fiber-rich foods also tend to have a low glycemic index, they will release sugar slowly and keep you going through even the busiest morning.

To get even more digestive benefits from your breakfast, pair it with a digestion-friendly drink like warm water with ginger, lemon, and honey or good old-fashioned coffee.

Here are a few of the best gut healthy breakfast options out there.

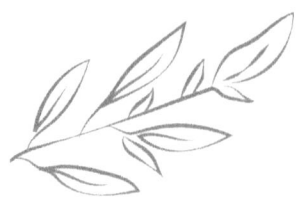

Fruity Oatmeal

Oatmeal is excellent for your gut (and many other things too), but adding chia seeds and fruit puts it in the realm of a gut health superfood. Adding yogurt, which is a probiotic, and honey, which has natural anti-inflammatory properties, makes for the perfect quick, easy, and delicious breakfast.

INGREDIENTS

1 cup of steel-cut oats, prepared according to package instructions
Two tablespoons of chia seeds
½ a cup of blueberries
1 tbsp yogurt (live culture)
Honey to taste

METHOD

Stir the chia seeds into the oatmeal. Top with yogurt and berries, and drizzle with honey to taste.

NOTES

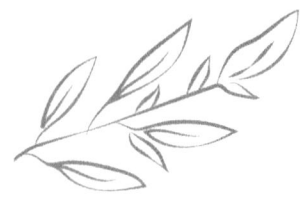

Florentine Cake Pan Omelet

Oatmeal is excellent for your gut (and many other things too), but adding chia seeds and fruit puts it in the realm of a gut health superfood. Adding yogurt, which is a probiotic, and honey, which has natural anti-inflammatory properties, makes for the perfect quick, easy, and delicious breakfast.
Here is how you can make a quick and tasty version of this dish, baked in a cake pan, so there is no fussy flipping to worry about.

INGREDIENTS

Two large eggs, whisked with a tablespoon of water or milk, and seasoned to taste
Olive oil to grease sheet pan
Two tightly packed cups of spinach, chopped
Two tablespoons live culture yogurt
Grated parmesan to taste

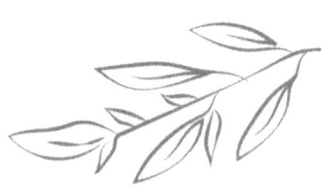

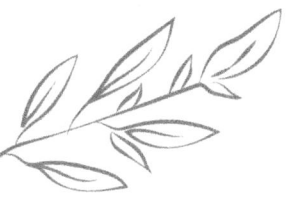

Florentine Cake Pan Omelet

METHOD

Preheat oven to 350F.
Lightly grease the bottom of a fixed base cake tin with olive oil.
Pour egg mixture into pan and place in preheated oven.
Wilt spinach in a pan with about a tablespoon of water. Spinach should be slightly softened but not completely limp. Add a little more water if required to prevent burning.
Keep spinach warm.
When eggs are just cooked on top, remove pan from the oven and invert onto a plate. The oil should allow the omelet to release easily.
Mix the yogurt and cheese into the wilted spinach, and spoon into the omelet.

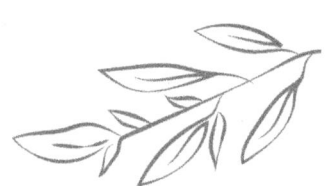

NOTES

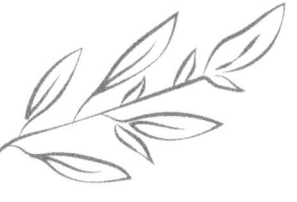

Oat Pancakes

Pancakes are the ultimate breakfast food, but when they are made out of refined flour with white sugar, they are not great for your gut. All of that changes when you add oats to the mix. The boost of fiber, protein, and cholesterol-busting power of oats makes your favorite breakfast a healthy choice for your body but still one of the tastiest options out there. These are thick, fluffy American style oat pancakes.

INGREDIENTS

1 cup rolled oats
1 cup almond milk
2 large eggs
1 tbsp butter
1 tbsp brown sugar
2/3 cups whole wheat flour
2 tsp baking powder
¼ tsp salt
¼ tsp cinnamon
Olive oil for cooking
Yogurt, honey, and fruit to serve

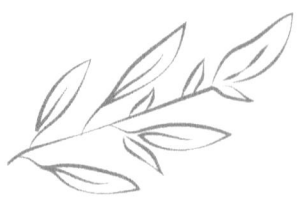

Oat Pancakes

METHOD

Mix the oats and the almond milk together in a bowl and leave to soak for ten minutes. This step is crucial to ensure that the oats are soft enough to make great pancakes.

Add the butter, eggs, and brown sugar to the soaked oats, and mix well.

Add the flour, baking powder, salt, and cinnamon and mix to combine.

Heat a little olive oil in a pan and drop spoonfuls of the pancake batter onto the heated surface. Depending on the size of the pan, you can cook three or four pancakes together.

Allow pancakes to cook until bubbles appear on the surface, and then flip to cook the other side.

Keep pancakes warm, and serve with live culture yogurt, honey, and high fiber fruit.

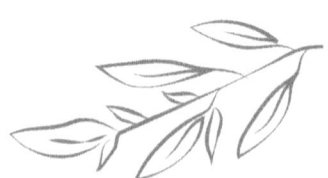

NOTES

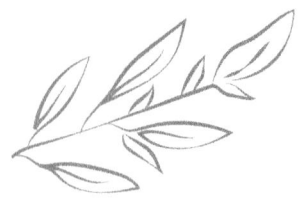

Quinoa Breakfast Bowls

Bowls are the best. They are easy to assemble, packed with all kinds of goodies, and in this case, the perfect gut-friendly combination of fiber, healthy fats, and protein. With just a little sauerkraut or kimchi to add a fermented flavor boost! This bowl recipe serves four.

INGREDIENTS

1 cup quinoa
1 3/4 cups low salt vegetable stock
Salt to taste
1 medium avocado
Lemon juice
2 medium green onions
2 tablespoons olive oil, divided
4 packed cups baby greens (kale, spinach, or any combination you like!)
4 large eggs
1 cup sauerkraut or kimchi if you like a little kick in your breakfast!
1 cup plain Greek yogurt

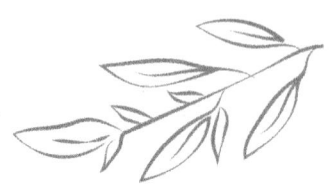

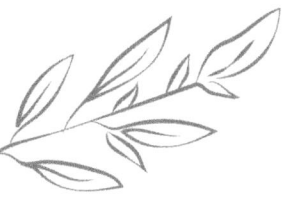

Quinoa Breakfast Bowls

METHOD

Rinse the quinoa, then place in a saucepan with the vegetable stock. Add salt and bring to a boil. Reduce heat and simmer till quinoa is tender or about ten minutes. Set aside, covered, to steam.

Heat half the olive oil in a pan and sauté the greens until wilted. Thinly slice the avocado. Sprinkle with a little lemon juice to prevent browning.

Divide the cooked quinoa between the bowls. Top with avocado slices on one side, kimchi or sauerkraut on another, and cooked greens on a third. Leave a space for the eggs.

Heat the remaining olive oil in a pan and lightly fry the eggs as preferred. (Over easy or sunny side up with a slightly runny yolk is delicious, but make sure you use pasteurized eggs.)

Top each bowl with an egg and enjoy!

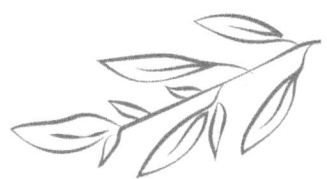

NOTES

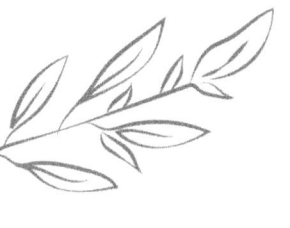

Kefir, Raspberry Ginger Smoothies

If you love smoothies, then you will be very happy to know that with a few tweaks, you can turn a mostly healthy smoothie into a gut health boosting wonder. Better yet, this mixture of kefir, berries and spice tastes great too.

INGREDIENTS

2 cups unsweetened almond milk
2 ½ cups frozen raspberries (or other berries of your choice)
1 packed cup baby spinach
3/4 cup plain kefir (or live culture yogurt if you prefer)
Juice of ½ lime
1" piece fresh ginger, peeled and coarsely chopped
Honey to taste

METHOD

Pour all ingredients into a blender.
Blend for about two minutes until smooth.
Pour into glasses. Serves two.

NOTES

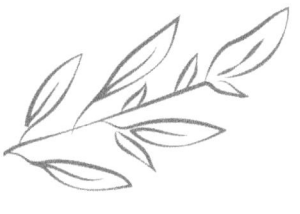

Breakfast Sweet Potatoes

If you thought sweet potatoes were only for roast dinners, think again. These sweet and delicious root vegetables make a fabulous fiber-packed breakfast. Even better, they are easy to make, and, topped with yogurt, a little maple syrup, and some nuts, they're super tasty too!

INGREDIENTS

1 small sweet potato or yam (scrubbed and with a few holes poked into each side with a fork)
Plain, live culture Greek yogurt
Maple syrup
Chopped unsalted nuts

METHOD

Preheat oven to 375F.
Place sweet potato on a baking sheet, and bake for 40 to 50 minutes, or until the point of a knife pierces the potato easily. Remove potato and allow to cool for a few minutes.
Cut a cross into the top of the sweet potato, place two fingers on each side of the cross, and press slightly to open up the flesh. Top with yogurt, drizzle with maple syrup and sprinkle with chopped nuts.

NOTES

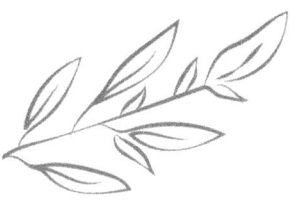

Whipped Cottage Cheese Toast

Whipped cottage cheese with stewed fruit on whole grain or seed loaf toast doesn't sound like a gut-healthy breakfast, but it is proof that just because food is good for you, that doesn't mean it can't be delicious. Make sure you look for cottage cheese with live cultures or substitute extra-thick live culture yogurt.

INGREDIENTS

1 cup of cottage cheese (makes enough for four slices of toast)
½ cup frozen fruit of your choice
¼ cup water
Honey to taste
Wholegrain bread or seed loaf, toasted

METHOD

To whip the cottage cheese, place it in a blender or food processor, and blend for one minute. The resulting mixture is light, fluffy, and more like ricotta than plain old cottage cheese.
Set aside.
Place the frozen fruit in a small saucepan with honey and the water. Cook over a medium heat until the liquid has dissolved, and the fruit is soft.
Spread toast with whipped cottage cheese (or yogurt), top with stewed fruit, and add a little drizzle of extra honey if preferred.

NOTES

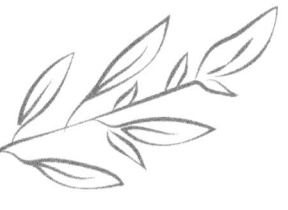

Coconut Chia Pudding with Fruit

Pudding for breakfast? That already sounds like a win. But when you add in the fact that this pudding doesn't need any cooking, you are onto a sure thing. Make this pudding the night before, and all you will have to do in the morning is choose and slice your fruit. Makes four servings of pudding.

INGREDIENTS

1 cup full fat coconut milk
¼ cup chia seeds
1 tbsp peanut or another nut butter
2 tbsp maple syrup
1 tsp cinnamon
Chopped fruit, blueberries, sunflower seeds, raisins, or shaved coconut to top (making your own mix is half the fun!)

METHOD

Mix everything except the fruit and toppings together.
Cover, and refrigerate overnight, or until the pudding is set (usually a few hours)
Top with your choice of fruit, berries, seeds, and other topping options, and serve.

NOTES

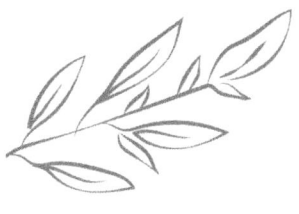

Wholegrain Apple Waffles

Waffles feel like a super indulgent breakfast, and they usually are. But by swapping the white flour out for whole-grain and adding grated apple, you can add a fiber boost that is great for your gut. If you top your waffles with yogurt, honey, and blueberries, you'll get probiotics and more fiber too.

INGREDIENTS

2 large eggs
2 tbsp oil
½ cup unsweetened applesauce
½ cup shredded/grated apples
½ tsp vanilla
½ cup cashew or almond milk
1 ½ cups whole wheat white flour
2 tsp baking powder
2 tsp ground cinnamon
¼ tsp salt

METHOD

Mix eggs, oil, and applesauce.
Add grated apples, vanilla, and nut milk, and mix well to combine.
Stir in flour, baking powder, cinnamon, and salt.
Heat a waffle iron. Grease lightly or as directed by manufacturer.
Spoon waffle batter into waffle iron and
follow directions to cook until done.
Serve hot waffles with yogurt, blueberries, and a little honey, or sauté more apples with a bit of oil and brown sugar and use to top yogurt.

NOTES

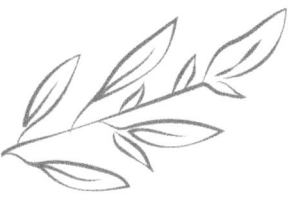

Breakfast Burritos

If you like a little Tex-Mex flavor in your breakfast, these breakfast burritos are the perfect choice. Substitute white flour tortillas for whole-grain and add lots of veggies to the mix to get a whole lot more fiber!

INGREDIENTS

Whole wheat tortillas
½ chopped onion
1 medium tomato, peeled and chopped
½ jalapeno, seeded and chopped
1 tbsp olive oil
Salt to taste
½ cup canned beans, rinsed and drained
½ cup cooked and cooled brown rice
Chopped cilantro/coriander
Squeeze of lime
½ avocado, diced
Scrambled egg
Live culture yogurt

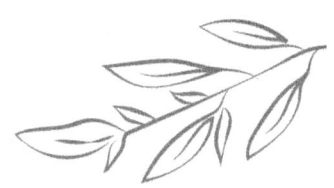

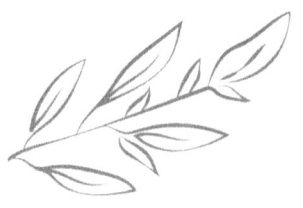

Breakfast Burritos

METHOD

Sauté onion in a little olive oil with salt to taste.
When onion is translucent, add tomato and jalapeno
and cook until soft and cooked through.
Stir in beans and cooked rice.
Lay one tortilla on a plate.
Spoon some of the bean, rice, and vegetable mixture into the
center of the tortilla, leaving one space at the bottom for folding.
Top with a layer of scrambled egg, and then add avocado, lime,
cilantro, and yogurt. Do not overfill!
Fold the bottom edge of the tortilla up and over the filling.
Fold one edge in to cover filling, and then fold the other over.
If preferred, lightly toast in a pan with a panini weight,
flipping to toast both sides.
Serve with a little hot sauce on the side if preferred.

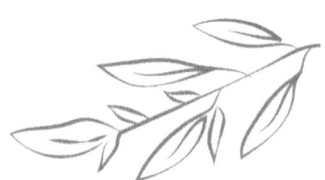

NOTES

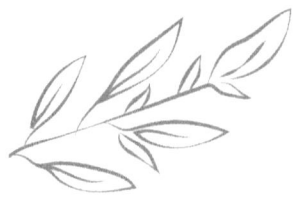

Salmon & Asparagus Frittata

It might sound decadent, but a salmon and asparagus frittata is actually good for your gut! Salmon has healthy omega-three fats, and asparagus has lots of fiber and probiotics. Eggs, of course, are a great, easy to digest source of protein, and yes, it does all feel just a little fancy. But you deserve it! Serves four.

INGREDIENTS

1 palm-sized salmon filet, lemon juice, dill, and salt to taste
½ small onion, finely chopped
1 clove garlic, chopped
1 tbsp olive oil
½ bunch asparagus, trimmed and cut into 1" pieces
¼ cup water
4 large eggs, whisked
Salt and pepper to taste
Grated parmesan to serve

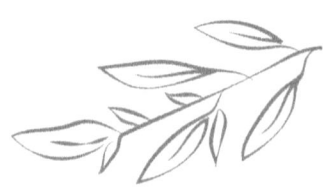

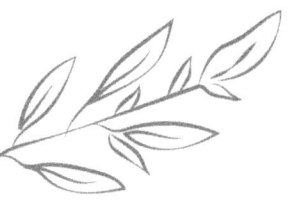

Salmon & Asparagus Frittata

METHOD

Preheat oven to 350F.
Poach salmon in a little water with lemon, dill, and salt. Remove from heat and set aside to cool.
Heat olive oil in an oven-safe cast iron pan.
Sauté onion until just translucent, then add garlic and asparagus.
Pour water into pan and cover to steam over a medium heat, stirring occasionally.
Flake the salmon, removing any skin if present.
When the asparagus is tender, and the water has evaporated, sprinkled flaked fish into pan, distributing fish and vegetables evenly, with spaces in between.
Pour whisked and seasoned eggs over vegetables and eggs.
Cook for a few minutes over a medium-low heat to allow the bottom of egg mixture to set.
Place pan into the oven, and bake for about 6-10 minutes, or until the top of the egg is set.
Cut into wedges, plate, and sprinkle with parmesan cheese.

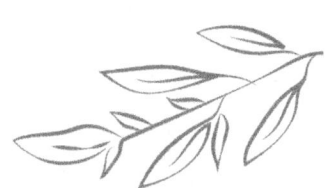

NOTES

LUNCH & DINNER

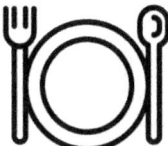

Gut healthy meals have lots of vegetables, fermented foods, smelly cheeses, lean protein, and warm spices. So, while you might be worried that you won't have anything to eat, you will actually be surprised at just how many delicious options you have that will also do wonders for your digestive system.

Most of the recipes we have featured here are also very easy to do, so they are perfect for days when you don't have the time or inclination to spend hours in the kitchen.

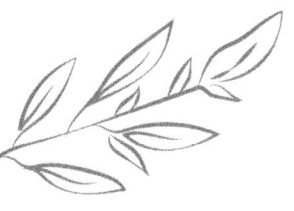

Pea Soup

Peas are packed with fiber and antioxidants, plus they taste great. Paired with spices and served with a swirl of kefir or yogurt, with some toasted whole-grain bread for dunking, they are also great for your gut.

INGREDIENTS

1 onion, chopped
Olive oil for sautéing
2 cups frozen peas
1 tbsp lemon juice
Chopped mint
Chopped parsley
2 tsp salt
1 tsp cracked black pepper
4 cups vegetable stock
Yogurt or kefir and toasted sunflower seeds, to serve
Whole-grain toast

METHOD

Heat oil in a heavy-bottomed saucepan.
Sautee onion until translucent.
Add peas to the pan and stir fry for a few minutes.
Add lemon juice, herbs, and seasoning, and stir fry for another minute.
Pour vegetable stock over vegetables, lower heat, cover, and simmer for 15 to 20 minutes.
Remove from heat and puree with an immersion blender to desired smoothness. Adjust seasoning.
Serve with a swirl of kefir or yogurt, a sprinkling of sunflower seeds, and toast squares to dip.

NOTES

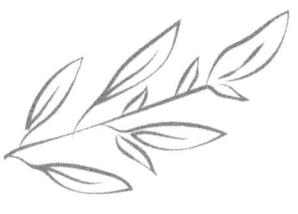

Thai Red Chicken Curry Soup

You might have heard that spicy food is bad for your gut, or the rumors that they cause ulcers and other gut health problems. The good news is that that is not true. The better news is that spices are great for your gut and general health. When you team them up with healthy fats, high fiber vegetables, and brown rice, they become a tasty way to do something great for your digestive system.

INGREDIENTS

1 can coconut milk
1 cup chicken broth or stock
3 tbsp red Thai curry paste (you may need to vary this based on the type you use!)
2 tbsp brown sugar
1 tbsp fish sauce
1 large yellow onion, diced
3 garlic cloves, minced
2-inch piece ginger, minced
1 cup broccoli florets
2 carrots, sliced
2 boneless, skinless chicken breasts
1 cup cooked brown rice to serve
1/2 cup roasted peanuts, chopped cilantro, beansprouts, and lime wedges to serve (optional)

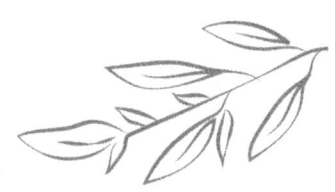

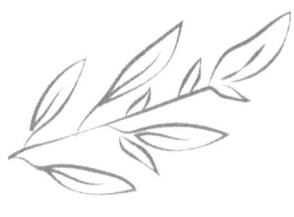

Thai Red Chicken Curry Soup

METHOD

Heat a small amount of olive oil in a heavy-bottomed saucepan, and stir fry onion, carrot, and broccoli until slightly softened.
Add chicken to pan and stir fry for a few more minutes, until it loses its pinkness. Add garlic and ginger and stir fry until fragrant and stir in brown sugar.
Add stock and coconut milk to saucepan, reduce heat and simmer gently to combine all the flavors.
Serve over cooked brown rice with your choice of peanuts, cilantro, beansprouts, and or lime wedges.

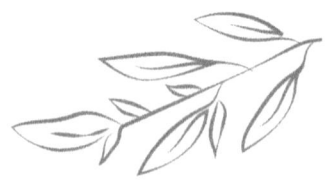

NOTES

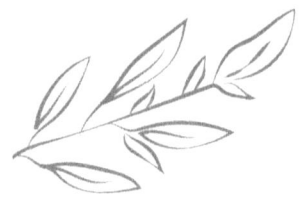

Chicken & Broccoli Salad with Miso Dressing

This warm salad is served over brown rice and dressed with miso features lean protein and tons of fiber, courtesy of the brown rice, and broccoli. Miso is not only tasty and packed with vitamins, but it is also a fermented food, and that means it is excellent for healthy gut bacteria.

INGREDIENTS

½ cup brown basmati rice, cooked
1 skinless chicken breast
1 cup sprouting broccoli
1 spring onion, cut diagonally
1 tbsp toasted sesame seeds
1 tsp miso paste
½ tbsp rice vinegar
½ tbsp mirin
½ tsp grated ginger

METHOD

Poach chicken in a little salted water or chicken stock.
Set aside and cool.
Steam the broccoli until tender.
Mix miso, rice vinegar, mirin, and ginger together for dressing.
Slice cooled chicken across the grain into thin
(1/2 cm or ¼ inch slices).
To assemble, place rice on a plate or bowl. Top with broccoli and chicken. Drizzle with dressing and sprinkle with sliced spring onions.

NOTES

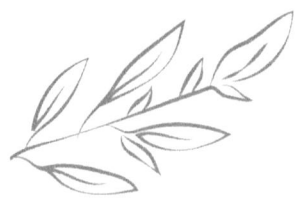

Spicy Korean Pork & Kimchi Soup

Kimchi is a wonderfully spicy Korean fermented cabbage condiment that is both a probiotic and packed with fiber from the vegetables. Combined with lean pork and cubed tofu, it is a great gut-healthy lunch or dinner that tastes like it shouldn't be good for you at all! In fact, this is a deliciously different take on Chinese hot and sour soup.

INGREDIENTS

1 tsp vegetable oil
100g pork tenderloin, cut into slices
½ small brown onion, thinly sliced
1 garlic clove, minced
¼ tablespoon finely grated fresh ginger
1 small carrot, peeled, chopped into 1.5cm pieces
2 cups chicken stock
½ cup kimchi, drained and coarsely chopped
½ tbsp gochujang
½ tablespoons soy sauce, plus extra to taste
100g silken tofu, cut into 1" cubes
½ teaspoons sesame oil
Thinly sliced green onions to serve

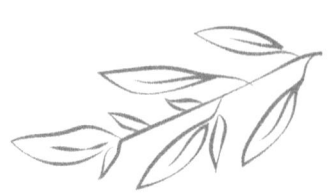

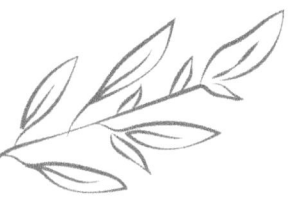

Spicy Korean Pork & Kimchi Soup

METHOD

Heat vegetable oil in a saucepan or wok.
Add pork slices and stir fry until lightly browned.
Add onion, garlic, and ginger and stir fry until the onion has softened (about two minutes.)
Add the carrots, chicken stock, kimchi, soy sauce, and gochujang, cover and simmer for about 40 minutes or until the pork is tender.
Add the tofu and heat through. Season with additional soy sauce, sprinkle with chopped green onions, and serve.

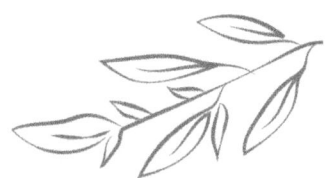

NOTES

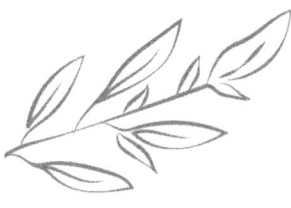

Mexican Rice & Bean Bowls

These Mexican inspired bowls are made with gut-friendly brown rice and black beans, topped with a little spicy chicken, vegetables, and live-culture yogurt. Add a little hot sauce for an extra kick, and sprinkle on a little shredded cheese for extra flavor (but remember that cheese is not great for digestion, so be sparing!)

INGREDIENTS

½ cup cooked brown rice
½ cup canned black beans, drained and rinsed
1 skinless chicken breast
1 tbsp reduced salt taco seasoning
1 tomato, chopped
½ small onion, thinly sliced
½ avocado, sliced and drizzled with lime juice
Chopped coriander
Live culture yogurt
Small sprinkling of cheese and hot sauce to taste

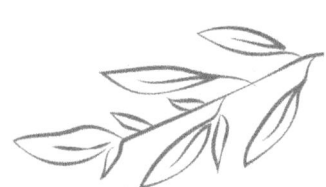

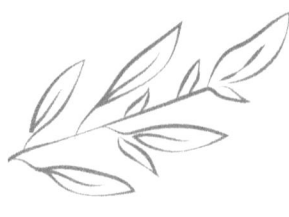

Mexican Rice & Bean Bowls

METHOD

Place the chicken in a saucepan with a little water, taco seasoning, and beans. Cover and cook, turning chicken occasionally until it is cooked through. Remove chicken and set aside to cool.
Cook beans with remaining water and seasoning until water is almost completely cooked away.
Shred chicken.
Place warm rice in a bowl, top with shredded chicken and beans. Add tomatoes, onions, and avocado to the bowl, then finish with chopped cilantro and yogurt.
Sprinkle a little cheese onto the bowl and add hot sauce to taste.

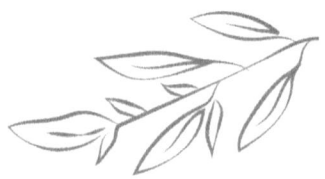

NOTES

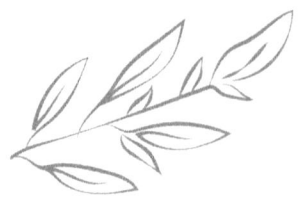

Sweet Potato Cottage Pie

Cottage pie is fantastic comfort food, but white potatoes without their skins are not great for gut health. Add more vegetables to your meat mixture and swap the white potatoes for sweet, and you have a dish that is hearty and good for digestion! Serves 4.

INGREDIENTS

1 tbsp olive oil
1 large onion, chopped
2 garlic cloves, chopped
2 medium carrots, grated or diced
2 tbsp fresh thyme leaf
1 lb extra lean ground beef
½ cup red lentils
1 parsnip, diced
2 tbsp plain flour
2 cups reduced-salt beef stock
2 medium potatoes, diced
2 large sweet potatoes or yams, diced
½ cup 0% plain probiotic yogurt
Ground nutmeg
green vegetables, to serve

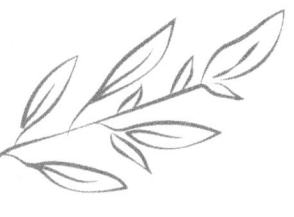

Sweet Potato Cottage Pie

METHOD

Heat oil in a heavy-based saucepan. Add onions and garlic and stir fry over medium heat until fragrant and softened.
Season to taste.
Add carrots and thyme and stir fry for one or two minutes.
Add ground beef, stir fry, breaking up lumps,
and continue cooking until beginning to brown.
Add lentils, parsnip, and flour to the pan, stir to combine, and then add the stock a half a cup at a time, stirring to combine between additions. Cook until the sauce is thickened, taste and adjust seasoning, then set aside.
Cook the potatoes and sweet potato in salted water until a knife pierces them easily.
Drain the potato mixture, and mash with yogurt.
Pour meat and vegetable mixture into an oven dish, top with potato and sweet potato mixture, and sprinkle with nutmeg.
Grill/broil in the oven until the top of the dish just starts to brown.
Serve with green vegetables.

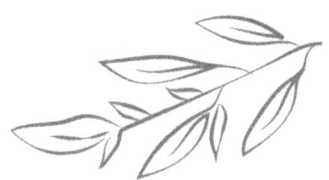

NOTES

Quick & Easy Kedgeree

This mildly spiced and delicious dish was originally popularized by the British in India. But this version takes all the best elements of that original dish and gives it a gut-healthy makeover with more fiber, a few extra vegetables, and of course, those wonderful gut-friendly spices. Serves 3-4.

INGREDIENTS

2 tbsp olive oil
leaves from 6 spring onion, finely chopped
½ tsp ground turmeric
1cm length of fresh ginger, grated
1 cup frozen peas
1 cup brown rice, cooked
4 eggs, hardboiled and roughly chopped
About 1 cup cooked, smoked, and flaked fish (salmon or mackerel are great for their Omega 3 content!)
salt and pepper to taste
chopped fresh coriander leaves

METHOD

Heat oil in a heavy-based saucepan.
Stir fry spring onions and peas until onions are slightly softened and fragrant.
Add ginger and turmeric, and then add cooked rice and stir well to combine.
Mix in flaked fish and boiled eggs, season to taste, and sprinkle with chopped coriander to serve.

NOTES

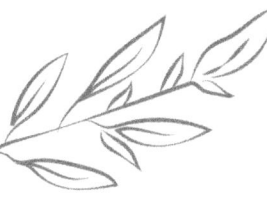

Wholegrain Reuben Sandwiches

Everyone needs a go-to meal for when they really don't feel like cooking, and the Rueben sandwich has many good gut health things going for it. By switching out the bread and making a few other little tweaks, you can increase its gut benefits. Serve with a salad with leafy greens and sliced, unpeeled green apples for added crunch.

INGREDIENTS

2 slices of whole-grain bread
Plain live culture yogurt for spreading
Dijon mustard
Slices of pastrami or corned beef
1 slice of low-fat Swiss cheese
½ to 1 cup of sauerkraut, well-drained

METHOD

Spread bread with yogurt, and drizzle with a little Dijon mustard. Lay slices of pastrami or corned beef on one side of the open sandwich and place the slice of cheese on the other side.
Add a thick layer of sauerkraut to the sandwich and close. Lightly grease a frying pan, and then place the sandwich in the pan to toast. Turn when lightly golden brown and repeat on other side. Remove from pan, slice, and enjoy with a crunchy green salad.

NOTES

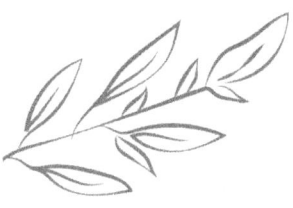

Roasted Vegetable Salad with Baked Salmon

Vegetables are fantastic for gut health, particularly those that are slightly woody, like asparagus. This wonderful salad and salmon combo can be baked on the same sheet pan for a lazy dinner that requires virtually no cleanup! Lightly dressed with a lemony sauce, it is a warm dish that still feels a lot like summer.

INGREDIENTS

Asparagus, trimmed and cut into 2" pieces
Zucchini, cut into 1" rings
Cubed butternut squash (cubes should be about 1")
Canned chickpeas, rinsed and drained
Cherry or grape tomatoes
Olive oil
Salt and pepper
Salmon fillet
Lemon juice, dill, salt and pepper, and olive oil for dressing

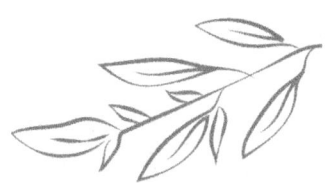

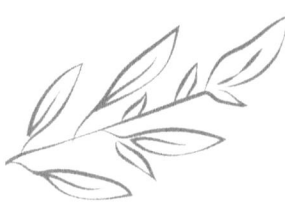

Roasted Vegetable Salad with Baked Salmon

METHOD

Preheat oven to 350F.
Toss vegetables in a little olive oil, and then season with salt and pepper. Place on one side of a baking sheet.
Lightly season salmon and place on the other side of the sheet.
Bake for 20 - 30 minutes, checking salmon to make sure it does not dry out. If salmon cooks before vegetables are tender, you can remove the fish and set aside while the
vegetables continue to cook.
Remove vegetables from the oven and combine in a bowl.
Mix lemon juice, dill, salt and pepper,
and olive oil to make a dressing.
Place fish on top of vegetables, drizzle with dressing, and serve.

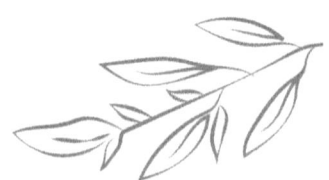

NOTES

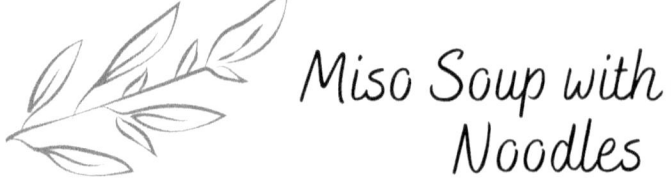

Miso Soup with Soba Noodles

Miso is a fantastic fermented paste packed with flavor and also happens to be very gut healthy. Soba noodles are made with buckwheat, so they have a low glycemic index and more fiber. Add plenty of vegetables and a few traditional flavorings, and you have a soup that tastes great and is gut healthy too! Serves 4

INGREDIENTS

4 cups vegetable stock
2 tsp instant dashi powder
2 tbsp mirin
1 tbsp soy sauce
2 carrots, peeled, thinly sliced
1 small daikon radish, peeled, thinly sliced
¼ lb halved shiitake mushrooms
2 tablespoons white miso paste
½ lb firm silken tofu, cut into 1/2" pieces
1lb soba noodles
Baby spinach leaves, shredded, to serve
2 teaspoons white sesame seeds
2 teaspoons black sesame seeds

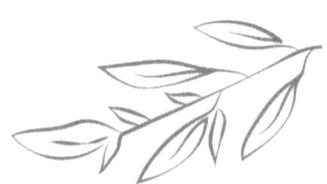

Miso Soup with Soba Noodles

METHOD

Place stock and 1 cup water in a saucepan and simmer over a medium heat.
Stir in mirin, soy sauce, dashi (if using).
Add carrot and daikon and cook for five minutes, then add mushrooms and cook for another five minutes, or until vegetables are all tender.
Add the miso and mix into stock with a whisk, then add the tofu to heat. Do not boil.
Divide noodles among bowls, pour over soup stock, and divide vegetables between bowls. Garnish with shredded spinach and sesame seeds.

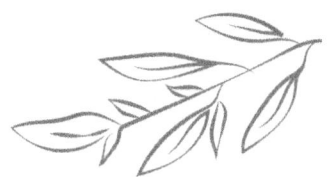

NOTES

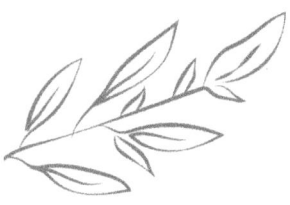

Lentil & Vegetable Dhal

Dhal is an Indian dish that is usually a chickpea or lentil curry with a delicious thick spicy sauce with additional vegetables. Legumes are great for your gut, and adding vegetables boosts the fiber content of this dish. Spices are great for your gut, and if you serve this with a spoon of live culture yogurt, you can add some probiotic power too.

INGREDIENTS

1 tbsp olive oil
1 red onion, finely chopped
2 garlic cloves, crushed
2 tsp fresh ginger, grated
1 tsp ground turmeric
1/2 tsp chili powder
1 cup split lentils, rinsed, drained
3 vine-ripened tomatoes, coarsely chopped
1 potato, peeled, coarsely chopped
2 teaspoons brown mustard seeds
2 sprigs fresh curry leaves
Brown rice and live-culture yogurt, to serve

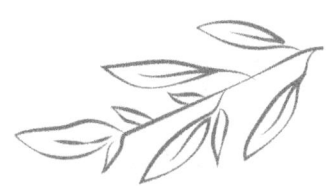

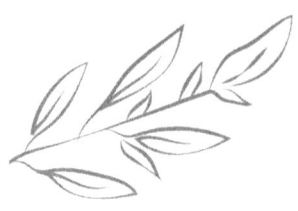

Lentil & Vegetable Dhal

METHOD

Heat oil in a heavy bottom saucepan.
Add onions, garlic, ginger, and spices, and stir fry over a medium heat until softened and fragrant. Be careful not to burn garlic or ginger!
Add tomatoes, potatoes, and lentils, along with 4 cups of water. Simmer gently for about 30 minutes, or until lentils are very soft.
Heat another tsp of oil in a small pan and fry the mustard seeds and curry leaves until fragrant, then stir into the lentil mixture.
Season dhal to taste.
Serve dhal over rice, with yogurt, to take a little of the heat off and add some probiotic goodness!

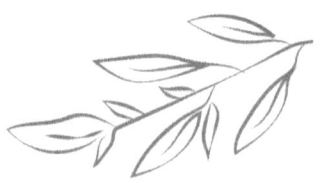

NOTES

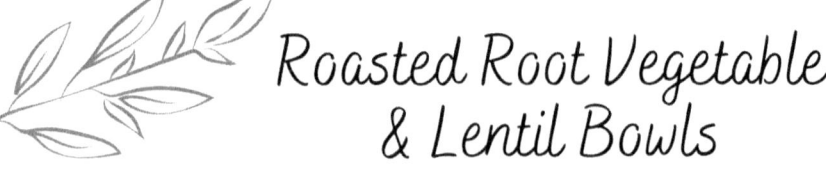

Roasted Root Vegetable & Lentil Bowls

Lentils are a great choice as a meatless protein substitute, and they contain fiber too. Root vegetables are fantastic for gut health, but when they are slow-roasted, they taste like they should be bad for you! Add a spoonful of plain live culture yogurt to get a probiotic boost too.

INGREDIENTS

Lentils
1 ½ cups water
½ cup lentils
1 tsp garlic powder
½ tsp ground coriander
½ tsp ground cumin
¼ tsp ground allspice
¼ tsp salt
2 tbsp lemon juice
1 tsp olive oil

Vegetables:
1 tbsp olive oil
1 clove garlic, crushed
1 ½ cups roasted root vegetables (cube, toss in olive oil and seasoning, and roast at 350F until softened and browned on edges)
2 cups chopped kale
1 tsp ground coriander
½ tsp ground pepper
¼ tsp salt
2 tbsp tahini
Fresh parsley

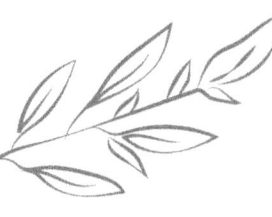

Roasted Root Vegetable & Lentil Bowls

METHOD

Combine all lentil ingredients in a saucepan and cook, covered,
over a medium heat until lentils are tender,
about 25 to 30 minutes.
Uncover and allow to cook a little longer,
until water is mostly evaporated.
Drain any remaining liquid.
Heat oil in a skillet, add roasted vegetables and kale. Sprinkle in
spices and seasonings, and cook together until
vegetables are warm and kale is wilted.
Serve vegetables over lentils,
topped with tahini and yogurt (optional.)

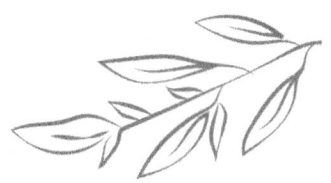

NOTES

Healthy living isn't restrictive, it's healing. Your health is something worth fighting for.

Unknown

SNACKS

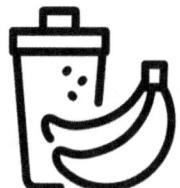

One of the biggest food misconceptions out there is that snacks are bad. Snacks are actually a great way to keep your metabolism working at its peak and keep your blood sugar levels steady. The problem is most of us are snacking on refined carbs with lots of saturated fat, salt, and sugar. None of those things are good for your gut. So, get rid of the chips, pretzels, and commercially baked muffins, and choose some of these gut-friendly alternatives.

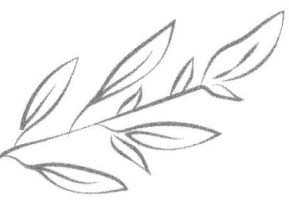

Hummus & Crudités

Hummus is one of the best snacks out there, and it is really easy to make your own. Chickpeas have fiber and protein, and when you add in some spices and fiber-rich vegetables for dipping, it's a perfectly satisfying snack!

INGREDIENTS

1 can chickpeas
¼ cup lemon juice
1 medium clove garlic, roughly chopped
½ teaspoon salt, to taste
½ cup tahini
2 to 4 tablespoons water, as needed
½ teaspoon ground cumin
1 tablespoon extra-virgin olive oil
Celery sticks, cucumber sticks, baby carrots, and other vegetables to serve

METHOD

Place all ingredients except the vegetable dippers in a food processor, and pulse until smooth.
Taste and adjust seasoning, serve with vegetables to dip.

Note: you can vary the hummus' flavor by adding sun-dried tomatoes, herbs, or roasted garlic to the mixture before blending.

NOTES

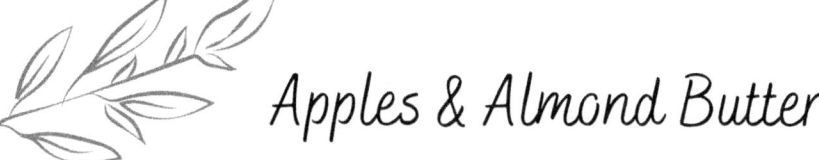

Apples & Almond Butter

This recipe is not even a recipe since there's really no preparation involved.
Simply slice your favorite type of apple (Granny Smith are ideal) into thin wedges (leave the skin on for extra fiber) and dip into natural almond butter. It is the perfect blend of creamy and crunchy and fiber and protein, with some healthy fat thrown in for good measure.

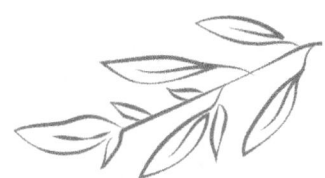

NOTES

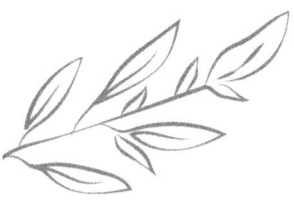

No-Bake Fruit & Oat Balls

If you have some time to make some healthy snacks ahead of time, these oat and fruit balls are the perfect sweet treat to keep in the fridge for up to a week, and they're fantastic for your gut, so there's zero guilt involved!

INGREDIENTS

2/3 cup dried apricot
¼ cup oats
¼ cup desiccated coconut
2 tbsp sunflower seed
1 tbsp sesame seeds
2 tbsp dried cranberries
3 tbsp protein powder or natural peanut butter
1 tbsp chia seeds

METHOD

Place apricots and oats in a food processor with 2/3 of a cup of boiling water. Puree together, scraping the sides of the blender.
Scrape the oat and apricot mixture into a bowl.
Toast the coconut, sunflower, and sesame seeds in a dry pan over a low heat.
Stir toasted coconut and seeds, cranberries, protein powder or peanut butter, and chia seeds into the apricot mixture.
Chill in the fridge.
Roll mixture into small balls, and place in small paper cupcake wrappers in a sealed container.
Will keep in the fridge for up to a week.

NOTES

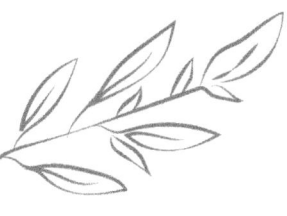

Wholegrain Banana Muffins

Another make-ahead snack option, and one that you can freeze and thaw in the microwave! These muffins have healthy seeds and fruit that pack a fiber-rich punch.

INGREDIENTS

1 ½ cups self-raising flour
¼ cup quinoa flour
¼ cup brown sugar
2 tbsp flaxseeds
1/3 cup mixed pumpkin and sunflower seeds
2 large ripe bananas
2 eggs, lightly beaten
1 cup live culture yogurt
1 tablespoon olive oil
1 punnet blueberries

METHOD

Preheat the oven to 350F.
Place 8 paper muffin cups in a muffin pan.
Mix all the ingredients except the blueberries to combine.
Stir in the blueberries, then spoon the mixture into the muffin cups.
Bake for 25 to 30 minutes, or until lightly golden.
Serve warm or cold.

NOTES

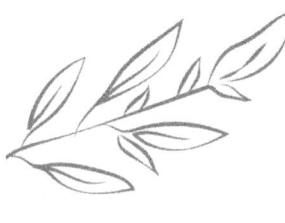

Sweet Potato Fries with Yogurt & Sweet Chilli Sauce

Another very quick and easy snack option that requires very little prep, this idea uses ready-made sweet potato oven fries. Prepare according to the package directions, and then serve with plain live culture yogurt and your favorite sweet chili sauce on the side for dunking. The fiber of the sweet potatoes paired with the live culture yogurt makes this a gut-healthy snack, even if it tastes like it is a cheat meal!

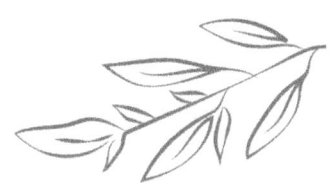

NOTES

JUICES & SHAKES

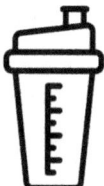

Commercial juices and smoothies are usually more sugar and salt than anything worthwhile for your gut. But that doesn't mean that they can't be part of a gut-healthy diet.

These juice, smoothie, and shake ideas are easy to make at home and the fresher you can have them, the better! These juices, smoothies, and shakes are made by blending the ingredients together, so we have just listed the ingredients for you.

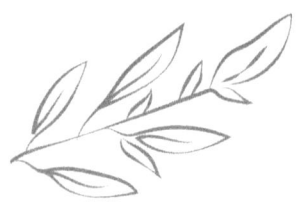

Juices & Shakes

PURPLE SMOOTHIE

3/4 cup coconut
or almond milk
2 cups purple kale (or regular
kale, although you will
not get the dramatic color!)
1 frozen banana
1 cup frozen blueberries
1 tbsp avocado
¼ tsp probiotic powder

GREEN SMOOTHIE

3/4 cup unsweetened coconut
milk
3 stalks red kale
3 stalks dinosaur kale
½ cup frozen mixed berries
¼ tsp probiotic powder

VEGGIE JUICE

2 cucumbers
1 green apple
1 lemon
1 inch ginger root
2 stalks kale
Fresh herbs of your choice
¼ tsp probiotic powder

CINNAMON STRAWBERRY SMOOTHIE

1 ½ cups almond
½ avocado
1 cup kale
1 cup frozen strawberries
¼ teaspoon cinnamon
5 drops vanilla extract

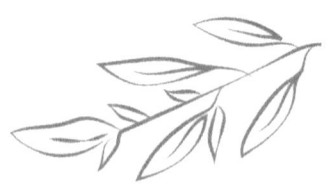

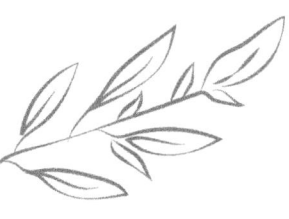

Juices & Shakes

PINA-COLADA BANANA

1 cup frozen pineapple chunks
½ large frozen banana
½ cup water
½ cup coconut water
¼ cup packed
fresh parsley leaves
2 tbsp avocado
1 tsp fresh grated ginger
¼ tsp probiotic powder, optional

CELERY JUICE

2 lbs celery washed, soaked, and chopped
2 large cucumbers washed, soaked, and chopped
1 large navel orange washed, soaked, and chopped
½ lemon

WONDER JUICE

1 small apple
3 medium carrots
½ beet
1 small lemon
1 medium cucumber
4 celery sticks
½ cup parsley
Fresh ginger to taste
2 tsp apple cider vinegar

BANANA PRUNE SMOOTHIE

2 cups unsweetened almond milk
2 tbsp almond butter
6 prunes
1 tsp cinnamon
1 small ripe banana

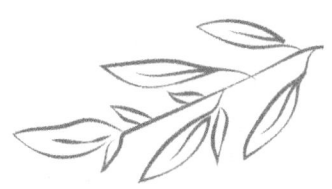

NOTES

Smoothies, juices, and shakes are a great way to get a meal or snack on the go, and it's actually very easy to make gut healthy drinks. Choose live culture yogurt or kefir, thin with herbal tea if necessary, and add frozen fruit or berries. A few green vegetables or some nut butter are great additions, and you can try endless different combinations to find your favorites.

If there is ever any doubt about what drinks you should be choosing, water and green tea are always safe choices, but as you can see, there are endless options! So, invest in a blender and a juicer, and use your favorite fruits and vegetables to drink the rainbow!

A Word on Alcohol

When you think of alcohol, you probably don't think about your gut too much, but while it's true that alcohol may have more direct effects on other parts of your body, there are some gut-related issues you need to know about.

The first is that alcohol has many empty calories in it, which means if you are trying to lose weight, and you have more than a few drinks a week, you are making it more difficult for yourself.

The other thing you should know is that alcohol contains a lot of sugar, and sugar, as we know, is very bad for your gut and the bacteria that live there. If you do drink alcohol, stick to medical professionals' quantity recommendations, and if you need to detox your gut, make sure that you eliminate alcohol while you do.

2 WEEK MEAL PLAN

Hopefully, you will have realized that eating a gut-healthy diet does not have to be bland or boring. In fact, adding herbs, spices, and yogurt-based sauces into the mix makes meals tasty as well as great for your gut.

However, if you still need a little inspiration, we've put together a sample two week menu for you that you can vary as needed. This can help you to stick to a gut-healthy diet as long as necessary to get everything working as it should.

Sample Two Week Menu - Week 1

DAY	BREAKFAST	LUNCH	SNACK	DINNER
Monday	Chia pudding with fruit.	Wholegrain Reuben sandwiches.	Home made trail mix (toasted coconut, mixed seeds & nuts, dried fruit.	Miso soup with soba noodles.
Tuesday	Kefir, raspberry ginger smoothie.	Quinoa salad.	Hummus & crudites.	Lentil & vegetable dhal.
Wednesday	Whipped cottage cheese toast.	Kedgeree.	Apple slices with almond butter.	Grilled chicken salad with kimchi and quinoa.
Thursday	Wholegrain apple waffles.	Mexican rice & bean bowl.	Cottage cheese on wholegrain crackers.	Miso soup with soba noodles.
Friday	Florentine cake pan omelet.	Pea soup.	Wholegrain crackers with cottage cheese and tomato slices	Reuben sandwiches.
Saturday	Salmon and asparagus frittata.	Lentil & vegetable dhal.	Mixed nuts and seeds and a small apple.	Curried butternut and coconut milk soup with wholegrain toast
Sunday	Oat pancakes.	Grilled chicken breast with roasted asparagus and tomatoes.	Hummus & crudites.	roasted vegetable salad with baked salmon.

NOTES

Sample Two Week Menu – Week 2

DAY	BREAKFAST	LUNCH	SNACK	DINNER
Monday	Florentine cake pan omelet.	Pea soup.	No bake fruit oat balls.	Kedgeree.
Tuesday	Whole grain toast with egg and half an avocado.	Mexican rice & bean bowl.	Frozen banana with dark chocolate.	Lentil & vegetable dhal.
Wednesday	Overnight oats	Thai red curry chicken soup.	Hummus & crudites.	Roasted vegetables with baked salmon.
Thursday	Chia pudding	Lentil & vegetable dhal.	Cottage cheese on wholegrain crackers.	Pea soup.
Friday	Strawberry banana smoothie.	Zucchini noodle salad.	Mixed fruit salad.	Backed fish with sweet potato.
Saturday	Whole grain apple waffles.	Waldorf salad with grilled chicken.	Mixed nuts and seeds and a small apple.	Spicy Korean pork & kimchi soup.
Sunday	Oat pancakes.	Miso soup with soba noodles.	No bake fruit oat balls.	Sweet potato cottage pie.

NOTES

Remember when your body is hungry, it wants **NUTRIENTS**, not calories.

Unknown

4

BONUS: EXERCISE

We all know that exercise is vital to our general health, but it is even more important for our digestive health. In fact, while scientists don't know precisely how, exercise has been proven to improve the gut microbiome in mice and in people.

Exercise also improves blood flow and muscle tone, which helps the intestines to do their job more efficiently. While you don't want food to move through your digestive tract too quickly, you do want it to make the journey with a reasonable amount of efficiency, and when it doesn't, you will find that things start to get backed up.

This book is not an exercise book. There are lots of those out there. This book is about easy, natural ways that you can improve gut health, treat common gut problems, and support the treatment of not so common ones. So, since the research shows that exercise is excellent for both the digestive tract's bacterial and muscular elements, it would not be complete without some tips on how you can easily incorporate gut-healthy exercise into your life.

Bloated? Get Moving!

Yes, the last thing you feel like doing when you are bloated is to move too much. Or at all. But all the research shows that that is exactly when you should get moving.

Because exercise has a beneficial effect on gut flora, if that is the reason for the bloating, moving will help get your gut flora moving and doing their thing to keep everything moving along. It will also physically help gut mobility, which will help to get whatever is causing you to feel discomfort through the system faster.

Exercise and gut health specialists recommend 30 minutes on a treadmill or stationary bike, or even a brisk 30-minute walk, to get everything moving.

The Best Exercises for Gut Health

If you are not a big fan of exercise, there is some good news: most gut health experts recommend low impact and low-intensity workouts, especially if you aren't fit.

High-intensity workouts can be extra hard on the gut, especially if you don't have strong core muscles to keep everything where it should be.

If you don't already work out regularly, your best bet is something a little less frantic, such as:

- Stationary biking or cycling
- Walking, golf, or yoga
- Swimming or water aerobics
- Strength training or weightlifting
- Crunches (they target the core muscles, which is great, but

make sure you do them correctly and don't overdo it when starting out!)

This is particularly important if you are suffering from constipation, which is likely to make you not want to move at all. Do something slow and gentle, but do something, because it will help to solve the problem.

When you have solved the problem, add a little higher impact exercise like dancing, tennis, or aerobics classes. These will help to tone up your muscles, which will improve your overall and specifically your gut health.

Build Up to It

Exercise is good, but stress is bad. If your workouts are too intense and make you feel worse, you won't look forward to them, you will stress out, and that will have a negative impact on your gut.

No one should ever go from 0 to 100 overnight when it comes to exercise, but that is particularly true if you have a gut sensitivity. Take it slow, don't push yourself too hard, but try to be consistent. It is better to do 20 minutes of moderate exercise a few times every week than to try to cram a month's worth into one day.

Breathe Intentionally

It may sound like some sort of new-age stuff, but there's been some research done that intentional breathing, and focusing on your abdomen when you do, can have a beneficial effect on your gut health and help you destress. Mindful breathing isn't exactly exercise, but it is a physical step you can take to support your gut.

Not Immediately After Meals

No matter what exercise you do and how often you do it, you should remember your parent's advice about swimming – give it some time after meals before you leap right in.

If you already have gut sensitivity issues, working out right after eating won't make you feel better. It will definitely make you feel worse. In fact, if you can time your workouts to happen just before you're supposed to eat, then wait a few minutes before you do, you will feel a whole lot better!

Check with Your Doctor

We won't go into any more detail about exercise in this book, except to say that if you don't usually exercise, and particularly if you have been diagnosed with a gut-related condition, you should always check with your doctor before starting any new exercise routine.

In most cases, exercise does nothing but good. Still, there might be rare occasions where a particular type of exercise is not recommended, and it is always best to check.

You should also remember that while a certain amount of muscle stiffness and soreness is to be expected when you start working out, if you have sharp or stabbing abdominal pain when working out, and it doesn't resolve itself within an hour or two, you should consult a doctor.

Yoga

Yoga is a great practice to include in your weekly health routine. It can be particularly helpful in improving gut health. This is because yoga is not only excellent for its fitness aspects but also incorporates breathing and elements of *"finding your calm"*. It can help you both de-stress and get in great shape. With the body control you gain, you will feel ready to conquer the world.

We wanted to add some simple poses and stretches you can perform to get a small taste of yoga. As an added benefit, these poses are said to help with digestion and detoxification of your gut.

Make sure not to push your body past any point you aren't comfortable with.

Knee to Chest

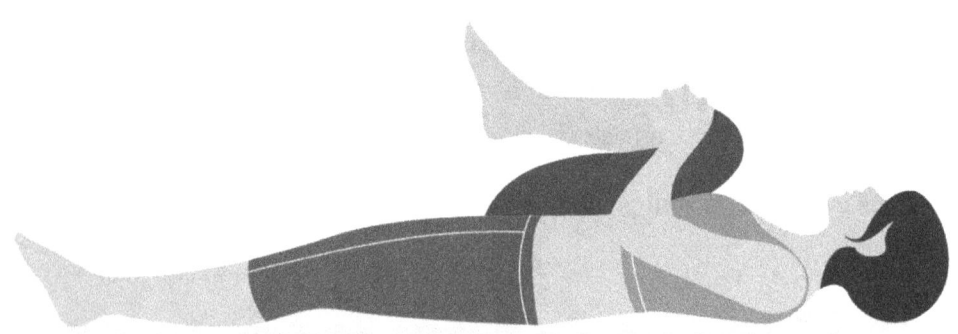

Get in a comfortable laying position on the floor with your feet stretched out and arms on your side. Keep your left food stretched out, and on an inhale, bring your right knee towards your chest. Clasp your hands around the top of your shin. Try to dive deeper into the stretch as exhale. Hold this pose for 5 to 10 breaths, then release, and repeat on the other side. This is an excellent pose for digestion and the release of tension.

Bridge

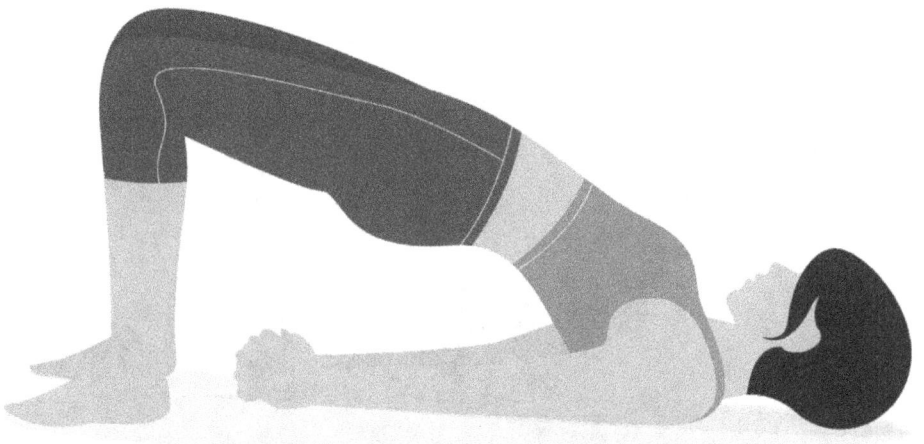

Get in a comfortable laying position on the floor with your feet stretched out and arms on your side. Bend your knees and bring your feet towards your butt. As you inhale, lift your hips toward the sky and lift your buttocks off the floor. Simultaneously clasp your hands below your pelvis. Keep your knees directly over your heels and hold this pose for 5 to 10 breaths. On the last exhale, slowly lower yourself out of the pose.

Leg Raise

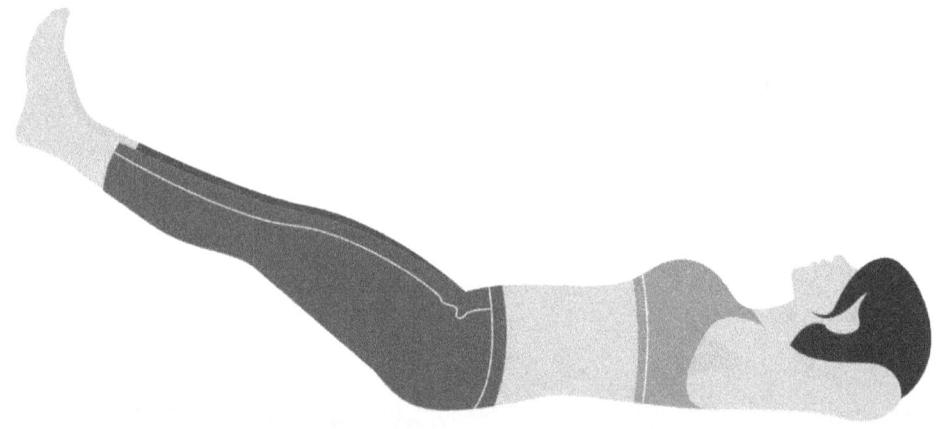

Get in a comfortable laying position on the floor with your feet stretched out and arms on your side. Turn your palms downwards against the floor, or clasp your hands behind your lower head. As you inhale, calmly raise your legs to around a 45-degree angle from the ground. Keep your legs straight as you hold this position for 5 or more breaths. On the last exhale, slowly lower your legs out of the pose. Never strain beyond your capacity.

Knees to Chest

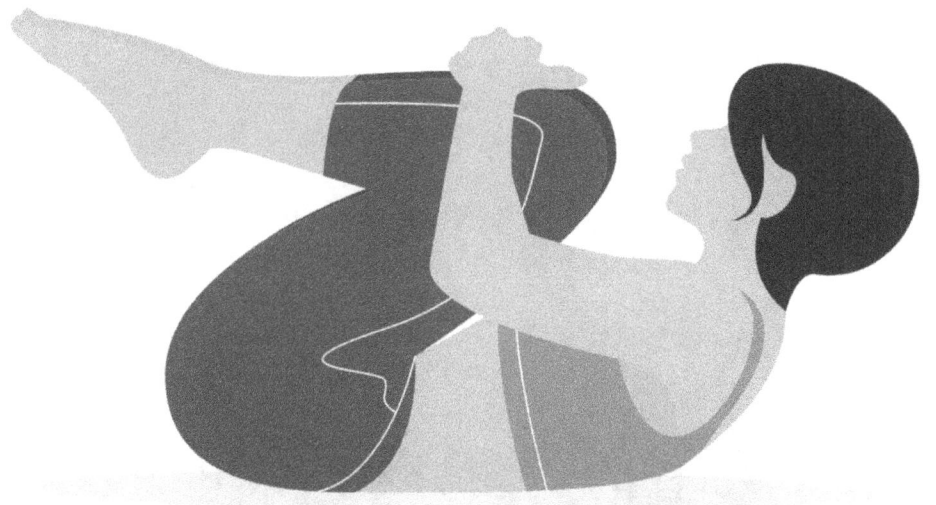

Get in a comfortable laying position on the floor with your feet stretched out and arms on your side. As you inhale, bring your knees gently towards your chest, and clasp your hands around the top of your shins. Hold this position for 5 to 10 breaths.
As you inhale, release the knees slightly, and as you exhale, hug them in more. If you are comfortable, feel free to gently rock from side to side and front to back to release tension.
You can also lower your head to the floor. This is an excellent pose for digestion.

Seated Twist

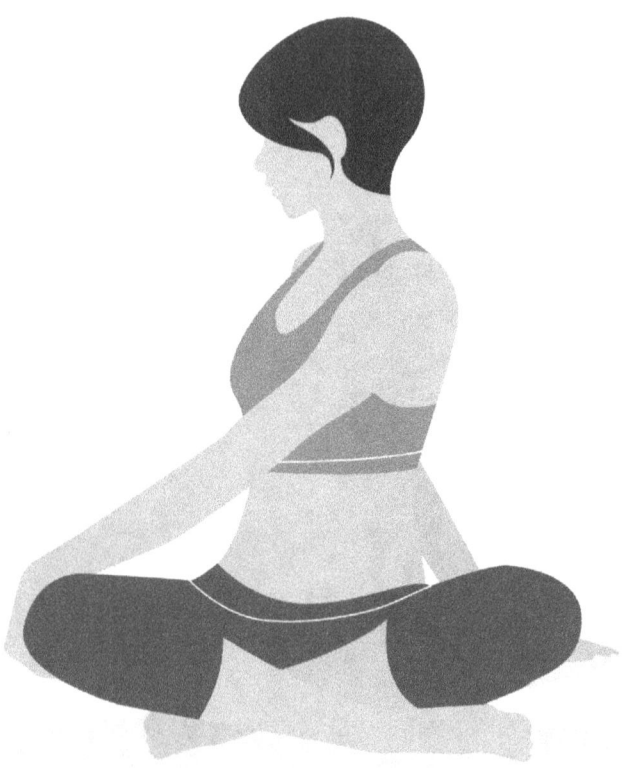

Get in a comfortable cross-legged seated position. Aim to sit with a tall spine and engaged core. With a deep inhale, raise your arms and lengthen your spine. On your exhale, slowly twist your upper body towards the right and look over your right shoulder. Place your right hand behind you and your left hand on your right knee. Stay in this pose for 5 to 10 breaths. Optionally and, if possible, lightly deepen your twist with each exhale. Once complete, repeat on the other side.

Side Body Stretch

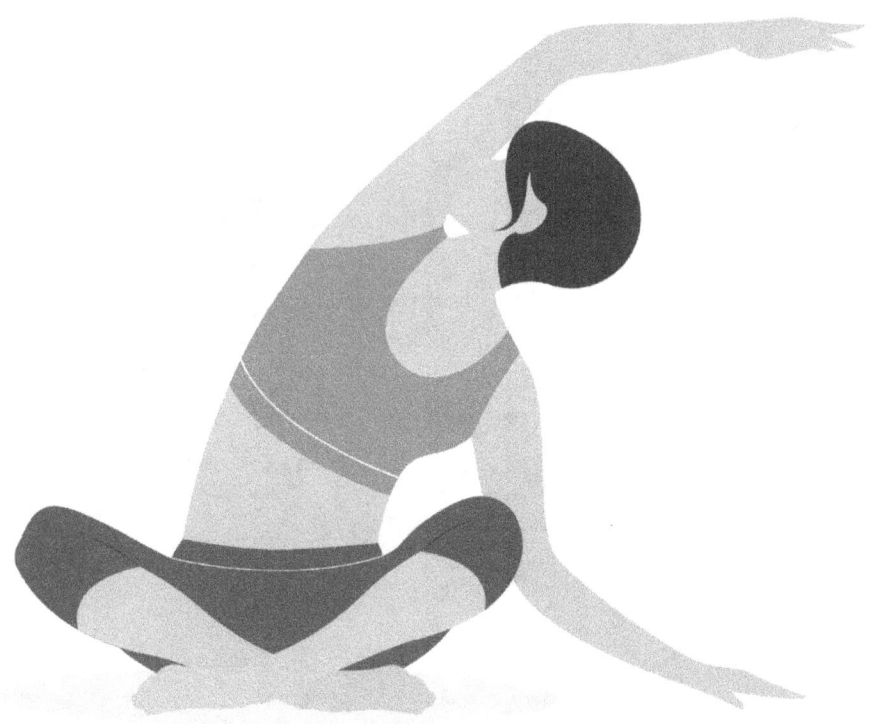

Start in a comfortable cross-legged seated position. Aim to sit with a tall spine and engaged core. With a deep inhale, raise your arms and lengthen your spine. On your exhale, place your left arm to your left side and shift your right arm and upper body to the left. Simultaneously shift your gaze upwards. Stay in this pose for 5 to 10 breaths. Once complete, repeat on the other side.

Thread the Needle

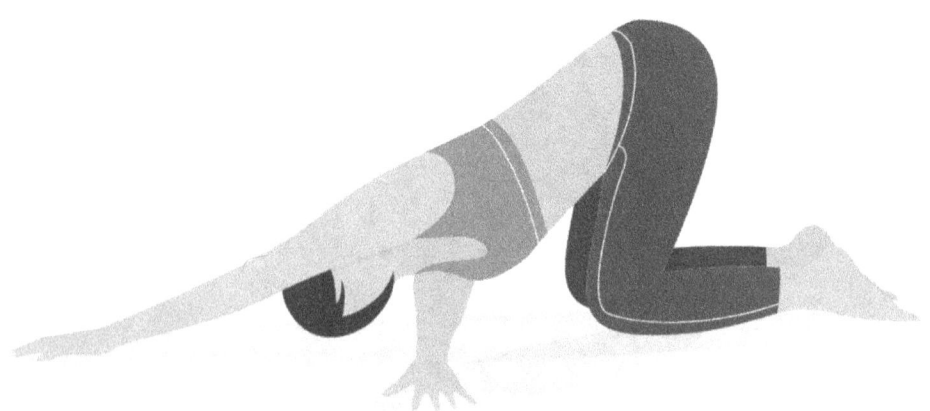

Get on your hands and knees, both shoulder and hip apart. Inhale. On your exhale, reach your right arm under your left arm. Continue by lowering your right shoulder and ear to your mat. Keep your hips in the air and maintain an equal weight in your knees. Hold this pose for 5 to 10 breaths. Once complete, release back to a neutral position on your hands and knees. Then repeat on the other side.

> If you think the pursuit of good health is expensive and time consuming, try illness.

Lee Swanson

AFTERWORD

It is hard to believe it's taken people so long to make the connection between good gut health and their overall wellbeing. After all, no other system is so integrally involved in fueling your body, or so literally intertwined with everything inside your body.

Poor gut health and an imbalance in the gut microbiome have been linked to everything from arthritis to cancer and heart disease, to poor immune function. It can make you absent-minded or moody, and it can cause you to gain weight and have trouble losing it. It may even be causing or worsening imperfections in your skin.

Your gut is both cause and effect when it comes to your overall health. When it is not working right, you will be sluggish, fatigued, more prone to get sick, and just feel generally unwell. When the rest of you is not well, particularly when you are stressed, one of the first places you will notice is in your gut.

There is no way to avoid or ignore the impact of your gut on your life and your health. The longer you try to ignore it, and eat foods that don't promote or actively harm your gut microbiome and make lifestyle choices that are bad for your digestive system, the more you will feel the effects.

Of course, the occasional gastrointestinal infection is unavoidable. Still, we hope that this book has shown you just how much your choices affect your gut health and how you can make easy changes that cost virtually nothing, but have a significant impact. These changes aren't big, complicated, or expensive, and you can start to make them today. In fact, the sooner you do, and the longer you stick to them, the better you will look and feel, and the only thing you will be left wondering then is why you didn't start sooner.

They say it takes twenty-one days to turn a new habit into a lifestyle, so if you plan to change your eating and exercise habits, try to commit to three weeks. If you can eat healthy and move more for that long, it will stop being a detox diet or a workout boot camp, and it will become part of your daily routine.

Even if you can't manage to eat well everyday or exercise for half an hour three times a week, every little thing you do, whenever you can, is a step in the right direction. Whether you're just trying to live a healthier life or have a diagnosed condition, if you take better care of your gut, it will take better care of you.

"

Create healthy habits, not restrictions.

Food Matters

THANK YOU

Thank you for reading this book and allowing us to share our knowledge with you.

If you've enjoyed this book, please let us know by leaving an Amazon rating and a brief review! It only takes about 30 seconds, and it helps us compete against big publishing houses. It also helps other readers find my work!

Thank you for your time, and have an awesome day!

**TRUST
YOUR
GUT.**

Unknown

RESOURCES

While we don't know everything about the gut, how it works, why it is so essential to so many things in our bodies, or how diet and exercise improve our gut and general health, there is ongoing research worldwide.

When you are looking for information on gut health (or anything else), the best places to look are always sites that are managed by medical organizations or medical journals, as they have nothing to gain by selling you miracle cures that cost a lot but don't achieve much.

These resources are some of the best in the world and a great place to start looking for more information.

Gut Health Organizations

Canadian Society of Intestinal Research

The Canadian Society of Intestinal Research or CSIR has been around since 1976, and is a registered charity dedicated to research and treatment of all kinds of gut health conditions.

https://badgut.org/

The World Gastroenterology Organisation

The World Gastroenterology Organisation (WGO) is an international federation of over 100 different organizations, all devoted to various aspects of gut health medicine and research. It's a great one-stop resource for all things gut related.

https://www.worldgastroenterology.org/

About IBS

IBS has been growing around the world for decades. About IBS is one of the organizations working to research what causes it and how it can be treated.

https://www.aboutibs.org/

Celiac Disease Foundation

About 1% of the population has celiac disease. The Celiac Disease Foundation is devoted to researching and treating this debilitating autoimmune condition. Here you can find resources related to getting a diagnosis, and when you have been diagnosed, advice on living with celiac, gluten-free eating, and more.

https://celiac.org/

Crohn's and Colitis Foundation

Crohn's and colitis are serious conditions that can have a profound impact on your health. The Crohn's and colitis foundation shares the latest research, treatment, and lifestyle tips for people who have these conditions, those that think they might, and their families.

https://www.crohnscolitisfoundation.org/

Gut Health Research Organizations and Papers

Many of the world's leading universities have departments devoted to gut health. Here are some must-read pages from institutions that share useful information about gut health:

John's Hopkins

5 Ways to Support Gut Health

John's Hopkins is one of the leading medical schools and research centers in the USA. This article is a collection of their top five findings related to supporting gut health.

https://www.hopkinsmedicine.org/health/wellness-and-prevention/your-digestive-system-5-ways-to-support-gut-health

Harvard Medical School

The Gut-Brain Connection

An article that references several research papers outlining the connection between the gut and the brain.

https://www.health.harvard.edu/diseases-and-conditions/the-gut-brain-connection

Oxford University

Gut Health Linked to Personality

An article citing research papers that details not only the connection between the gut and the brain, but the effect of the gut microbiome on personality.

https://www.ox.ac.uk/news/2020-01-23-gut-bacteria-linked-personality

Mayo Clinic

Examining the Role of Gut Microbial Composition and Function in Weight Loss

A detailed article referencing several studies that link gut flora to weight gain and the ability to lose weight.

https://www.mayoclinic.org/medical-professionals/digestive-diseases/news/examining-the-role-of-gut-microbial-composition-and-function-in-weight-loss/mac-20454980

US National Library of Medicine National Institutes of Health

Exercise Modifies the Gut Microbiota with Positive Health Effects

A report on the physical and bacterial flora effects of exercise on the gut.

https://www.ncbi.nlm.nih.gov/pmc/articles/PMC5357536/

National Institutes of Health

Gut Microbe Drives Autoimmunity

A report on how the composition of gut flora can trigger or worsen autoimmune conditions, including those not directly related to the gut.

https://www.nih.gov/news-events/nih-research-matters/gut-microbe-drives-autoimmunity

US National Library of Medicine National Institutes of Health

The Gut Microbiome and Its Role in Obesity

An article that outlines how the composition, diversity, and balance of gut flora could be causing obesity in some people, and how improving diet may help.

https://www.ncbi.nlm.nih.gov/pmc/articles/PMC5082693/

Journal of Medical Microbiology

Differences Between the Gut Microflora of Children with Autistic Spectrum Disorders and That of Healthy Children

One of many recent articles highlighting the difference in gut flora in children who have autism, and those who do not.

https://doi.org/10.1099/jmm.0.46101-0

Frontiers in Microbiology

The Gut Microbiome as a Major Regulator of the Gut-Skin Axis

A detailed study into the connection between gut flora and skin health.

https://www.frontiersin.org/articles/10.3389/fmicb.2018.01459/full

OTHER BOOKS BY BRITTNEY & CRAIG

- Liver Detox & Cleanse

To find more of our books, simply search or click "Brittney Davis" or "Craig Williams" on: www.amazon.com

www.ingramcontent.com/pod-product-compliance
Lightning Source LLC
LaVergne TN
LVHW012105070526
838202LV00056B/5631